Taking Back Your
Health *and* Happiness

Advance Praise

"Heartfelt and original. This book inspires people to look at causes of their suffering through a different viewpoint. People will learn about how to listen to their own bodies and know more about themselves. Healing the body is not just about taking pills, but achieving balance."

—**Tarah Pua**, MD, Gynecologic Oncologist,
New York Presbyterian Queens, NY

"Totally worth reading. Fierce, powerful, and absolutely breathtaking, this beautifully-written book that will sweep you away. It will captivate you from start to finish. I loved every word and highly recommend it! This book had it all—beautiful writing, beautiful story of each client, beautiful cover. This book is for people like me ready to move up to whole new level, to improve health and wellbeing. This is what I need…a high quality information and guidance towards optimal health. I learned a lot from this book."

— **Emy Avelino-Barba**, RN Riyadh, Saudi Arabia

"A story of spirituality and self-healing. Anyone who has ever been physically or spiritually ill will find solace in this book. This is a terrific guide for identifying one's mental bases of physical manifestations, establishing a plan of action for making a change, and overcoming obstacles to reach one's goal of healthy body and mind. An inspirational read."

— **Galina Borodulina**, MD, Anesthesiologist, New York

"Enlightening."

— **Marc Gregory Y. Yu**, MD, Endocrinologist,
Research Fellow, Joslin Diabetes Center, Boston, MA

"This book successfully harnesses the power of positivity! I learned and appreciated the guidance and wisdom of the CLEAR healing method. The author offers wonderful and holistic practical, medical, and spiritual stories weaved with personal journeys."

— **Niel Kenneth Jamandre**, Educator, Speaker, Philippines

"Reading the first two chapters itself is so moving, since I am a Filipino I can relate with Filipino values and all. The rest of the book is quite enlightening to read, especially to a person with high functioning depression like me. The book really is highly recommended and worth reading."

— **Lilibeth Munoz Cubillas**, Riyadh, Saudi Arabia

"Informative and comes from a realist's point of view. It doesn't sugarcoat and is an eye opener. It pretty much covers all the things we people often neglect. The content of the book is easily understood and is so relatable. That is why I highly recommend it for everyone to read. I hope this book reaches each corner of the world."

— **Kristie Caren Jimunzala**, RN Riyadh, Saudi Arabia

"This book is an inspiration and will give light to those who still cannot find the purpose of their lives, as well as for those who thought that they already know themselves. I believe that many people will be rescued from darkness."

— **Idah Gan Germo**, RN Philippines

"At some point in our lives we will experience the complete opposite of joy, peace and good living. During those cold prolonged moments where our health deteriorates and our soul shuts down, I wish we all had a bit of Marie Anne's advice with us, as she herself lovingly explains it in this empowering book."

— **Jose Murga**, New York

"Truly a masterpiece! Due to the demands of household and raising a toddler and a newborn, I said to myself, I didn't have time to read. But after reading the first part I just couldn't stop. It is an eye opener. I can totally relate to it. It opens up your entire senses and motivates you to become the better version of yourself. It teaches me to become more humane, more human to others, to be more forgiving to myself and to others. It enable me to open up to myself more and to others. Teaches me to become more holistic and God-fearing. As a whole, this book is a blessing. A motivator of life. Very uplifting! Very inspiring!"

— **Ma. Krizia Ledesma-Libre**, RN, New Zealand

Taking Back Your

Health

and

Happiness

Hope and Healing from Chronic Pain,
Fatigue, and Invisible Illness

MARIE ANNE
JUNE L. TAGORDA

NEW YORK

LONDON • NASHVILLE • MELBOURNE • VANCOUVER

Taking Back Your Health *and* Happiness
Hope and Healing from Chronic Pain,
Fatigue, and Invisible Illness

Published in New York, New York, by Morgan James Publishing in partnership with Difference Press. Morgan James is a trademark of Morgan James, LLC. www.MorganJamesPublishing.com

Disclaimer: The author does not assume any responsibility for errors, omissions, or contrary interpretations for the subject matter herein. Any perceived slight of any individual or organization is purely unintentional.

The information provided in this book does not intend to diagnose, cure, or treat any disease or medical illness. It is not to be used to replace medical and/or psychological services. As deemed necessary, please consult a physician, medical, psychological and/or psychiatric professional.

Stories in this book are based on true life experiences. Events were recreated from the author's recollections. Personal information may have been altered for privacy purposes.

Credits: Scriptures quoted from The Holy Bible, New Century Version, copyright 2005 by Thomas Nelson, Inc. Used by permission. All rights reserved.

ISBN 978-1-64279-593-6 paperback
ISBN 978-1-64279-594-3 EB
ISBN 978-1-64279-595-0 Audio
Library of Congress Control Number:

Cover Design by:
Rachel Lopez
www.r2cdesign.com

Interior Design by:
Bonnie Bushman
The Whole Caboodle Graphic Design

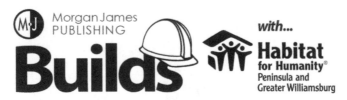

Morgan James is a proud partner of Habitat for Humanity Peninsula and Greater Williamsburg. Partners in building since 2006.

Get involved today! Visit
www.MorganJamesBuilds.com

This book is dedicated to my mother, Morita Lim, and my aunt, Sonia Lim. I love you both!

I am grateful and truly blessed for my beautiful mother, Morita Lim. Her passion, hard work, resilience, faith in God, and love for people have been my rock and have been a huge influence in my life. Thank you for being my greatest supporter.

I also want to thank the wisdom and support of my dearly departed aunt, Sonia Lim, who has been instrumental in the idea of writing this book, even after her death. She has been an inspiration, motivation, and driving force for me to bridge the gap between the physical, mental, emotional and spiritual aspects of self to those similar to herself. Thank you for shedding light on the path of my purpose.

Table of Contents

Foreword

A little over a decade ago I first met the author while attending a Healer School at Sedona Mago Retreat. After many years and twists and turns of fate the two of us were reunited, again in Sedona, when Marie Anne underwent a personal apprenticeship with me to become a spiritual intuitive reader and guide where I watched her further bloom into the embodiment of all that is goodness and compassion; an embodiment that was so natural to her that it made it clear that she was truly always meant to lead and care for many people who may be struggling here on this Earth.

When Marie Anne asked me to read her book and write its foreword, I couldn't wait to see what this intuitive healer with a nursing degree came up with... and again I watched the bloom grow bigger. Written with as much heart as mind, *Taking Back Your Health and Happiness* is an uplifting, informative, and charming read that outlines a truly holistic and compassionate approach to self-care healthcare based upon years of inquiry, experience, and personal implementation. It is with great pride that I have the opportunity to recommend this book to you.

—**Rebecca Tinkle** *is an award-winning author,*
American writer, and film producer.

Chapter 1
The Problem

OUCH, life! Why so rough with me? You may feel that life has not been easy for you. You often had to struggle to get to a better place. You have grown and learned to navigate many hurdles in life for a better future for yourself and your family. So, now that life is better than before, why does your body feel like crap? Why does it feel like something is wrong, be it headaches, back pain, joint pain, swelling, fatigue, insomnia, skin issues, or anxieties that cannot be explained?

You may be tired of being on all kinds of medications, trying to find out which works, seeing physicians and specialists, and awaiting diagnosis. It could easily affect your career or work, which you may have had to put on hold due to unmanageable pain, extreme fatigue, and invisible illness with unknown causes. Disappointments and frustrations can create an emotional toll on your relationships and can turn into depression. You may have tried turmeric or foods that help with inflammation, coenzymes, glutathione, and vitamins but are still living with unease and discomfort.

It is not easy when you have a life with many responsibilities and obligations. You may have grown up fighting your way up to have a better life for yourself and your family. You have always strived to be better and successful, educated and well informed, and taken many opportunities that came your way to provide a life of comfort for yourself and your family. You have been anything and everything that was needed, growing in strength, knowledge, and skills to get to a place of security and comfort.

Oftentimes with work, family, and relationships, you tend to put them ahead of yourself. You make many sacrifices such as sleep, time, and distance, such as being away from your family for long periods of time because you can see the future you are creating. This is what drives you to be resilient and strong. You are doing all this to have what you didn't have and to provide a more quality way of life for your family, especially for the future of your kids. Your kids are your number one priority, and you will do anything to make their life easier. You do not want your kids to go through any hardships or struggles like you did. You do not want your family to be lacking; you want the best you can give them.

As a younger you, sleeping less and working more, even skipping meals was a piece of cake. You may even have had more than one job. It was something you know you could handle. But as you get older, this changes. You grow less able to keep up with this kind of lifestyle. So sometimes, you adjust accordingly.

This way of life becomes a habit even when you have reached your goal for yourself and your family. Unknowingly, your way of life, accumulated thoughts, and emotions can subsequently stay with you and your body when they have not been processed through or let go.

This book will not touch much on the medical aspect of things and does not intend to diagnose, treat, or cure any disease or medical illness, but it will touch on the many possible sources of your physical unease and discomfort. There is a deep connection with what your body is feeling in relation to you as a whole.

You may have feelings of pain in a specific part of your body. Chronic shoulder pain and headaches are more common than you might think. Did you know that there are many types of headaches? There is one that is concentrated on the temples, one on the base of your head, one originating from the top of your head, and another could be your entire head. You may also have rashes, allergies, sensitivities, and even joint pains. Insomnia or difficulty sleeping may be a problem. Fatigue or persistent tiredness can also come up. You have probably seen one or more doctors or specialists who could not clearly explain your condition because your test results, assessments, and imaging results are showing nothing wrong. This can be very frustrating. You may be afraid that it could become something else or something worse if not resolved soon. It is very scary.

You may also feel like no one understands you and that people think that you are just making this up. You may feel misunderstood and that no one is on your side. At the same time, you do not really want to share this issue or issues with your loved ones or those closest to you because you do not want to burden them with what you are going through, even though deep down you wish you could tell them. This creates a heavy load for you to bear, but again, your loved ones come first for you, and you do not want them to have a difficult time. You might then decide to just keep things to yourself and not share what bothers you. This actually creates a strain on yourself and your relationships. It can create a rift and misunderstandings.

In time, these physical manifestations can affect your mood and your physical capacity to fulfill your work. You might be calling out sick often, which could be detrimental to your job. Either that or you push your body, which is already being stretched to its limit, to complete your everyday tasks and responsibilities.

You are tired of seeing one doctor or specialist after another and tired of trying all kinds of different medications to see what helps. You do not want to feel horrible and uncomfortable, which causes your anxiety. Being impatient, quick to anger, irritable, and moody dampens and creates a rift in your relationships with others, especially those you love. It may cause you to be cranky and unintentionally push your loved ones away.

You may be unable to fully share your heart because of your own ambivalent feelings about letting others in on your issues. Because of this ambiguous feeling, you are unable to clearly communicate your messages to those you love, thus creating misunderstandings. Not knowing how to approach you or how to help you can cause a lot of stress on you and your family. The key lies in *how* you communicate. As you read further, you will know the process to the "how" of communicating.

Chapter 2
My Story

Memories of my childhood bring about a sense of nostalgia. I remember being the one who always tried to make others feel comfortable and feel welcomed. I did not like seeing anyone feel left out. Growing up, I was very intuitive and a free spirit who enjoyed playing outdoors amongst nature. I'm told I was a very happy child who was naturally people-loving and effortlessly candid and funny.

As I grew up, I felt the need to achieve my family's expectations of me. Whenever I did well, congratulations needed no words, but whenever I made a mistake, there would be criticism to be better. Sometimes, it could be a form of punishment. Through this, I learned to be resilient and be a hard worker, but I also learned to become a perfectionist. I became very hard on myself whenever I made mistakes.

I was easily forgiving of others but not of myself. I would often hold on to blame and shame.

I grew up away from my mother and father because they had to work outside our country, the Philippines, to provide a better and more comfortable life for us. I often missed my mother, who I have a very close relationship with. It was always a celebration whenever my mother came to visit me because that was the only time I felt that I could openly and freely be myself.

I also became confused at some point in my upbringing. Whenever I did not follow instructions on what was expected of me, I would be punished. When asked why I did not follow, whether I answered with an explanation or not, I would still be punished. It would either be, you are being disrespectful when you do not answer, or you want to fight back if you answer. It made me feel hopeless that no matter what I chose, I was always on the losing end. I became resilient when receiving beatings and punishments, fighting back tears even when I almost blacked out or had a bloody nose. I became fearful of asking permission and dreaded having to ask.

In years past, physical punishment was an acceptable form of discipline. And although my mother did not treat me this way, I was exposed to this way of life. Even at a young age, I vowed to never ever be like that to my own family or kids someday.

As a teenager, whenever I felt that I was not good enough, whenever I did not reach others' expectations, or at least what I thought was expected of me, I used to hit myself. I did not care if I got seriously hurt. I used to hit my head hard against the wall because I felt that no matter what I did, I was never good enough, even though I was among the top students in my class. Physical pain was something I could handle, but the emotional and mental pain were deeper. Thankfully, I found many ways to find meaning in life. I filled my life with what I enjoyed doing as my mother supported me in my interests.

At ten years old, my family reunited in New York, USA. However, within a year or two, my mother and father separated. I may have been the catalyst in having their relationship out in the open. At that age, I was highly intuitive and asked my father, "Dad, do you love Mom?" Without hesitation, he answered, "No." I remember the time that my parents had a heated conversation wherein my father wanted me to be present in the room to better understand their situation. I was in the middle of the room with my father on one end and my mother on the other end, seeing and feeling everything that transpired. Although I was still little, I could feel my mom's pain and anguish and my dad's aloofness and unhappiness. At that age, words did not have as much an impact on my understanding. It was the feeling I was getting that I understood more.

When my father left, I saw how hurt and in pain my mother was. Because I had a deep and close connection with my mother, I became angry with my father. I was just getting to know him too, as he and I did not communicate much when he was away. I completely shut him and his family out of my life. That was how angry I was. For some time, I even ended up having no trust in and hating men.

Fortunately, later on in life, I refused to give up on people's humanity and goodness, and I learned to slowly heal. Growing up, I've had uncles who have been constant in showing what care and love is. I was fortunate to have many uncles who in their own way have been there for me. I had an uncle best friend who was so supportive in my time of angst with my parent's separation. They have been consistent in showing me that men can be caring, loving, and can be trusted.

In my early college days, I had come to a peak in my life. I was at the top of my class, very well liked, a leader and a school officer, and a major member of the school club. I had everything I wanted, everything I needed, and everything I hoped for, but there came a time that I had a sense of something missing or lacking that was making me very sad and lost. I could not figure out what it was but that there is something wrong, even when everything seems to be just right. No one seemed to understand where I was coming from so I just kept that to myself, knowing I had to go through that for a reason. I had a strong faith in where God was leading me and decided not to focus on that feeling, only to find out later on that the feeling was a message as well. Looking back, I believe I went through a midlife crisis at a very early age. This was in the first two years of my college life. I was seventeen to eighteen years old at the time.

I was very busy in Nursing school, being in clubs, hanging out with friends, spending time with family, and fulfilling church responsibilities. I loved getting to know people and learning new things. However, being busy also meant sacrifices in sleeping or time for unwinding. This was also the time I had my first love relationship with a wonderful person. We were together for about four years and had plans for marriage. However, things did not work out and we broke apart. It was a very painful process for me. Recalling those moments of low, I would often wake up with bouts of uncontrollable tears and pain, having difficulty breathing while sobbing and crying. My chest would be so painful as I couldn't control my crying. It made me very exhausted. I watched TV series online almost all day long to get my mind off of the pain. I thought, "I know it's painful now, but you will be alright." My belief was that it would probably take me about two years to really heal and move on. This was about the time I started to take up yoga classes, back in 2006. Four months later, my mother gifted me to be part of a Healer's School program held in Sedona as a birthday present. She knew I loved healing and was interested in the program but did not have the funds. I was so thankful but also went to the program with a heavy heart and sadness. I knew I was going to learn techniques and principles of holistic energy healing but did not anticipate that it would also give me the space to have a real talk with myself. Sedona is a beautiful place that has a vibration that promotes healing. It always feels like I'm coming home. My experience was a cocoon of love and self-reflections. It was where I realized and experienced that healing does not have to take a long time, as I initially believed. Being clear helps in facilitating your own healing. Although there was still residual emotional pain, I knew with clarity that my decision was right and in alignment with my heart with regards to my breakup with my ex-fiancé. I saw clearly the difference between love and pain inside of myself that propelled me to inspire hope and readiness to ignite happiness in my life again.

Upon the start of my nursing career, I started working the night shift. I often had to go back and forth to adjust my days and nights to have a full day off. There was no such thing as a set sleeping time. I ate during the night and slept throughout the day. It was the opposite whenever I had two or more days off in a row. There were also many days when I did not get to eat on time or use the restroom for long periods of time due to work.

I have moved around in nursing units to find what fit better for me. I have taken care of many patients and their loved ones and wished to be able to help them more on an energetic level as much as they were being helped on the physical level. I have had patients who are in constant and chronic pain who are on multiple medications, hoping to have some normalcy and relief from constantly living with pain. I see the effect it has on their loved ones. I have also taken care of patients who underwent surgery due to cancers. I see the many similarities and the individual differences in their energy bodies as I help them regain their optimum physical health and also help their emotional body. Many times, I see the patients' families needing this support a lot more than the patients themselves. As I am able to see and feel energy more and more, I am aware of the deeper aspect of their overall well-being. Oftentimes, they are not aware and are not ready for such healing. When someone is not ready for help, the help you wish to provide will have resistance and not much growth will come out from it as compared to the one who is ready.

As a nurse and as a healer, I have always been physically active and energetically abundant. I'm known to be petite in frame but strong in strength. I also have a lot of energy to do many things and take on many projects or interests all at once.

With all these plus a high tolerance to pain, I did not even realize that I developed chronic shoulder pain and tightness. Working in stressful situations would often give me shoulder tightness, heaviness of the head, and headaches. Sometimes, I felt tired along with the headaches, thinking I just need rest. There were days when I would have a hard time falling asleep despite feeling extremely exhausted from the day's work and times when I get to sleep long hours but woke up feeling very tired. I even started to have rashes around my mouth that came and went on their own without any known triggers.

After two car accidents in 2016, it hit me how out of tune my body was despite my being physically active. I was given acetaminophen and prescription NSAIDs (Non-Steroidal Anti-Inflammatory Drugs), namely naproxen and ibuprofen, for pain along with baclofen which is an antispastic muscle relaxant. I also did many epidural and trigger point injections. Surgery was also advised on my neck, lower back, and right ankle. I had been told to either undergo surgery or live with my issues. Being a recovery room nurse, along with my own beliefs and feelings regarding my body condition at the time, I asked for second opinions about having surgery. Putting in consideration all these, I decided to opt out of surgery and recover as naturally as possible. I decided this because I knew that I was very sensitive to medications. I felt like a walking zombie when I took my medicine. I could not even remember almost half the day for three full days. The injections gave me a boost initially but then made me feel a little off afterwards, and the relief did not last long. I had seen an orthopedic surgeon, a spine specialist, a chiropractor, a pain management doctor, an acupuncturist, physical therapists, podiatrist, and massage therapists for help.

After some time, I was told that I no longer need to see them. However, the acupuncture was the one that gave me some relief with no side effects. I actually felt like a normal person, even if just for a few hours. Knowing I had to work more to pay for my acupuncture sessions, I decided to take all I learned throughout the years about looking in and listening to my own body. It took a lot of effort to find a way to realign, replenish, and gather energy due to my body's condition.

This forced me to look for ways that worked best for me. I had to take a long hard look at all aspects of my life, including whether or not my accidents were messages for me. The last one took me off of work for almost a year. I started to ask God and the universe, "Are you trying to tell me something?" I started feeling depressed and asked myself these questions, "Where do you want to be? What can you see yourself doing for the rest of your life? What would you like to be doing until your very last breath here on earth? Is what you are doing now what you want to do until the day you die?" This created a shift in how I lived my life. I became more mindful and aware of the messages my body and my environment were telling me. Through the pain, fatigue, and frustrations, I learned to figure out the healing process that worked best for me. I applied what I learned in dealing with my own chronic pain issues, depression, and frustrations, and this helped me find hope in taking back my life. Through this process, I found that I am able to choose how to live my life. I am so excited to share my process with you, as I gained so much more than I ever expected.

Chapter 3
The Process
(CLEAR Healing Method)

I became frustrated knowing that medications do work, but they often do not fit me well. Acetaminophen and ibuprofen alone already helps me fall asleep. I tried baclofen and it knocked me out for three days.

I was living through the day like a zombie, not even remembering half of what happened during the day. "I do not want to live like this," I hear myself say. I would rather have the pain over feeling apathetic and drugged out. I only took my medications because I could not handle the pain anymore and didn't know what to do with myself. I was either not getting enough sleep due to the pain or not getting quality sleep.

From that point on, with that experience and that knowledge about myself about medications not being a good fit for me in the long run, I became more proactive in learning more about my pain and why I got tired easily. I knew this was not me because I know myself to be a vibrant human being. Where did that bold and vivacious me go? What happened?

There's an article in the *New York Times* titled, *Why Your Cardiologist Should Ask About Your Love Life,* written by cardiologist Dr. Sandeep Jauhar about how diet and exercise are no longer the only recommendations for a healthy heart. We are in a culture and society focused mainly on the physical health. But you know that we are more than just our physical body. The culture of embracing the whole and not just the physical needs to be cultivated. This shift in mindset of embracing and including the other aspects of ourselves as part of our overall health can create our optimal well-being.

Going through the steps in this process opened up my mind, my heart, and my body… not just knowing but actually feeling the other aspects of myself. This was how I learned to manage my pain better without side effects of taking strong medications.

In life, there are steps you need to climb for growth and understanding. Like in school, you have to complete first grade first before you can move on to the second grade, and so forth. These are the 5 Steps to Healing in my process of transformation. It is called the CLEAR Healing Method.

The CLEAR Healing Method:

Step 1—Clear and Cleanse
Step 2—Listen and Feel
Step 3—Establish Action or Inaction
Step 4—Act to Inspire and Motivate
Step 5—Receiving—(Achieve, Accomplish and The Art of Receiving)

Clear & Cleanse is about clearing your mind and cleansing your body from all the clutters and heaviness that are holding you down.

Listen & Feel will share the messages of your body and help determine whether what you're hearing is just a noise of judgement or the voice of truth.

Establish Action or Inaction will show you how your decisions affect your mind and your body. You will find that they are related.

Act to Inspire and Motivate is about habits of being critical about yourself and becoming your own cheerleader and support.

Receiving—(Achieve, Accomplish & The Art of Receiving) shares how following through with your commitment to healing deserves celebration. Embrace all that is good and harmonious to your well-being.

In the following chapters, I will delve deeper and explain further each of the steps of the CLEAR Healing Method.

Chapter 4
The Promise

Having seen many doctors and specialists, taken all kinds of tests, and tried out many different kinds of pills, I will not be talking too much about the medical aspect of things or the type of diets you should be eating, as you likely already know as much as you can in that light already.

I want to share with you what helped me become closer to and know my body, hear its messages, and understand why I'm feeling what I'm feeling, plus what I needed to do when these messages came to me.

Before embarking on the journey of healing, I had to make a promise to myself. I made a commitment that no matter what it took, I would do my very best to achieve my goal, which was to learn more about myself so I could understand and heal. I decided that I would not stop no matter how hard it might become to grow into healing.

I knew that there would be obstacles and all kinds of things that would show up to try and steer me away from my commitment. I anticipated that I would be tested on my conviction to fulfill my promise.

I had to prepare myself physically, mentally, and emotionally to meet these obstacles. I had to prepare a mindset of will and determination. Know that there will be moments that you will get sidetracked, but that is normal. As long as you become aware of them, just step back onto your path and continue on to fulfill your promise to yourself. The awareness of what is important and knowing that you have stepped off your path is already a form of growth.

It is extremely important to create this sacred contract. This is an essential prerequisite to the CLEAR Healing Method. I use the word sacred because it is very personal and intimate. It is a commitment to yourself. Many times, we take for granted our own promises to ourselves as opposed to our promises and responsibilities to others, be it our work or job, our partners, our husband or wife, our children, and other things. We prioritize others over ourselves. We know we need rest, but we don't rest because we think that we have to do this and we have to do that. There's no time to rest. And you wonder why you're tired or you get sick! We often neglect to take care of ourselves because we are too busy taking care of other things. This pattern gets repeated so many times over that it becomes a habit. It becomes a normal part of our lives. Without thought, we go into the motions of what our body is used to and do what we think is normal. But in reality, this is not the norm. We are the ones that have made it our normal.

Why are other things more important than our health? In perspective, we should really be taking good care of ourselves so we can optimally take care of the other things that are important in our lives. When you become ill, you just stay home, feel miserable, hunker down, and sleep away, having no appetite and just feeling horrible. On the other hand, when you have optimal health, you can go for what you want. You can work, play, spend time with family and friends, and do so much more that your heart desires.

So why not invest the time and space to commit to your own growth and healing? This book will share with you a nonmedical approach. Note that it is important to continue to see your own doctor or specialists. They will offer you medical wisdom and knowledge about your situation and a different kind of clarity than the process that I am about to share with you.

Know that you are important enough. You deserve to feel the best that you can feel. It is your right to live your life fully.

Take that right and have the conviction to live that life.

"You have a right to your own body and your own life."

This statement is what we want to believe to be true but deep down are not living it. When you become ill and it persists, you go see the doctor. Then you wait and see what the doctor says and what they will prescribe for you. It can feel very vulnerable and frustrating, especially when they cannot give you a specific answer and when they are unable to diagnose what you are going through.

When this happens, I notice an unconscious shift of energy. I feel that when you ask for help, you give up the bulk of the responsibility over your own body to the physician or specialists or whoever you put as the authority over your ill body. There is a sort of energetic transfer of responsibility: Here is my body; figure out what is wrong with it and fix it, then I can take it all back. When you look at it in a different light, in actuality you are the one who is the best resource about your own body. You are the one who knows exactly how your body has grown up, where it has been, what it has gone through, and what you have been making it go through. You are the one who can best know your body, and you need to start paying attention because it is telling you something. You are the authority over your body and you need to acknowledge and validate that. Even when your body is sick, be aware that there are people who can help, but you are still the sole CEO or president of your own body. You have the most stake in your life, so it is important to be proactive in learning all aspects of yourself.

Know that you have power over your life. However things may be in your life right now, know that it is never too late. There never is such a thing as too late. Time does not discriminate. Only our perception of time and what 'too late' means to us create the stress within ourselves. We may feel the need to quickly catch up because time is running out, or we feel helpless with not taking the opportunity and the time has lapsed. It is never ever too late to grow and heal our wounds as long as you still have breath left in your body. We have a time limit in living our physical existence on this earth. So what better time than *now* to upgrade your life? The Now is always the best time to create the change you want in your life. It is the best time to move forward, to create, to heal, and to grow.

Why not now? Is your health and well-being less important than other things in your life right now? What is stopping you from living your life right now? Why wait to start living your life later instead of starting to live it now? If your body is already signaling to you that something is wrong and there is no explanation of what you are feeling, then why is *now* not the time to commit to knowing more about yourself and growing in the space of healing?

What are you afraid of? Is your fear greater than the possibilities of growth and healing? What have you got to lose? If anything, you will learn many things about yourself along the way. As humans, we are gifted with the power to create through our choices. We live the life that we live because of our choices.

Committing to knowing yourself for growth and healing is a choice. Choice is your power. You have the sole power to choose how to live your life. Choosing is significant in life. Whatever choices you make determine the life you live. Someone could have suggested or recommended this book to you, but ultimately, it was your choice that got you here, reading this book. Similarly, you get to choose whether you follow these steps or not. The question is: Do you choose to stay where you are right now and continue to feel the way you feel, or do you choose to commit to knowing yourself?

A sincere mind is needed to grow in the path of healing. Know that you may encounter many things and learn many things about yourself that could make you feel uncomfortable and uneasy. You might dig up or effortlessly remember many painful or bittersweet memories you might have from the past. Anything can happen. Know and trust that anything and everything that will come up is precisely what is needed, is part of the process, and is meant to be at that moment. Because you decided to grow and know more about yourself, many lessons will show up. Be open to any and all possibilities. The more you expand your mind, the more you will see and learn.

Be prepared for challenges, distractions, and temptations that will test the conviction of your choice. There will be highs and lows. Like a roller coaster ride, there are ups and downs, twists and turns, and even loops along the way. It's how you perceive the ride and the attitude you choose that will determine whether it will be a fun and enlightening ride or the most miserable and most horrendous time you will have. There will be scary moments and moments that might make you feel nauseous, but that is all normal. Know that it is the time when the most growth can occur if you choose to be open to it. On the upside, there will be moments of epiphany, a light bulb that will shine a clear understanding, and those times will be absolutely brilliant and enlightening.

Having a conscious connection with your body is important to hear what it is trying to tell you. Pain and fatigue are some of the indications that something is not balanced. Many times we take painkillers or sleeping pills right away. We shut away the messages of our body. The more we shut out our body, the more we distance ourselves from hearing what it is trying to tell us. We create a disconnect in our relationship with our body. Many of us have not been taught to listen to our bodies. I remember the times that I came home from work and would see blacks and blues on my thighs or hips or arms and not even remember exactly when and how I got them because I was too busy taking care of others that day. Throughout the day, I had bumped into the chair, the table, the bed, and the computer and just kept going. I remember waking up one day with a swollen and sprained thumb and could not remember where it happened or how it happened. It took some time to remember. I had to backtrack the memories of my day and remember that the night before, I had hurt it while moving a heavy box out of the hospital closet and had not even given it a thought.

While at work, I was so focused on taking care of my patients first that I got into a habit of tuning myself out. I had to relearn to be consciously mindful of being tuned in. That small event taught me how even the little things—like a small part of your body like a thumb— matter. You do not realize how your thumb plays a big role in your everyday life. How much more do our heart, our brain, our liver, our lungs and such? According to Aristotle, "The whole is greater than the sum of its parts." This was a clear example of that for me. Every part of you is important. Taking care of your being as a whole and not just bits and pieces of you is optimal in your well-being. It is a great reminder that it is essential to take care of yourself first as much as you value taking care of others.

There is a reason why you are here at this particular moment in time, just like it is not likely just a coincidence that you are reading this book. If this book is not meant for you, you would have stopped chapters ago or may not have even picked it up. However this book arrived in your hands, whether it was a gift or a recommendation or you just happened on it, there is a reason. I didn't think of circumstances this way before. But with everything I've been through, all the people I've met, the circumstances I have been in, the trainings that presented themselves, and the decisions I made—all those led me here, right now. I realize that all those experiences and precious moments are not coincidences at all. They were aligned to where they were meant to be and where I was meant to be at the time. They were my lessons, my teachers, my students, my trainings, and a product of my decisions. Those decisions led me to see a clear picture that everything I went through and everyone I interacted with were there with purpose. It cultivated me into who I am and where I am now. It has led me to learn about myself, grow into healing, and find my life's purpose.

In my journey of healing, I learned way more than I expected or ever imagined. It is liberating to finally see myself clearly. You may think you know yourself already, but once you sincerely commit to your own growth and healing, there is a sense of freedom and ownership. Healing, learning, and growing is an ongoing process. I learned to see and break away from the invisible chains and prison that I had put on and built around myself. Going through this process made me see that I was the one who placed that on myself. Seeing and acknowledging that helped me start to peel off layers and layers of what was holding me back from fully living my 100%. Living your authentic self can help release a lot of the blockages and baggage we are holding in our bodies.

In the bible, Jesus says, "Ask and you shall receive." Whatever you sincerely ask will present itself in front of you. It may not always come in the form that you expect, but it comes just the same. It is your choice whether to accept it or walk away from it. Again, it is your choice. The power of your choice.

This is a journey and a contract of "Me, Myself, and I." Get to know your body and create a close and healthy relationship with your own body. Just like in a relationship, your body being your partner, you need to have a proper conversation. You need to listen when it is complaining. If you know that you were not good to your body or have put it through rigorous terrain, you now have to woo or court it back to happiness, homeostasis, or its optimal state. Get to know your body and find out what is wrong, what it is complaining about. It is like a child throwing a tantrum, angry because you did not pay attention to him or her. You need to listen or he or she will make your life suffer in the form of pain, tiredness, insomnia, allergic reactions, headaches, etc. I could go on and on. You need to show your body that it is loved.

You need to be able to have a talk with your body and your spirit. With apology, gratitude and love, tell yourself:

"I'm sorry, my body! I'm sorry my truth, my spirit, my soul. I'm sorry for not paying attention to you and for taking you for granted. You have always been there for me, keeping up with me and my demands. I did not listen when you were trying to talk to me. I'm sorry for shutting you out in the past."

"Thank you for sticking it out with me, putting up with me, and hanging in there. I have put you through many things and yet you have always been loyal and ever present for me. I am here now, 100% present, as you have been for me. I hear you. Let us make this work. Please be patient with me as I need to come out of my habit of tuning you out and not listening. I promise to love you from here on out. No matter what it takes, I am choosing to know and grow myself to healing. I accept 100% the responsibility and ownership of my own body. I commit to being the authority of my life."
"I commit to loving you and all aspects of you!"

Chapter 5
STEP 1—Clear & Cleanse

The first step in the healing process is Clear & Cleanse. This means emptying the mind and cleansing the body. This is to help reset the body and the mind. It is akin to a computer, which you might have to restart because it is sluggish, stuck, slow, or overheating—just like when our bodies start to feel this way. It is also like cleaning up the house so that it will be easier to find what you are looking for. Let go and throw out the things that you do not need and keep the things that you need. Empty first so that you can fill it with whatever you choose.

For most of us, we are born with an innate ability to heal. Our body was built this way. For instance, when we fall and hurt our knees, when we get a scratch or a cut, we clean it. Whether we put medicine on it or not, it heals in a few days. You may notice that healing time may be quicker for some than others. In Western medicine, we talk about what is called WBC (white blood cells), also known as leukocytes, that help fight off infection and protect our bodies. They act as the soldiers of our physical body, fighting off and neutralizing irritants and foreign microorganisms that attack our body. They also create antibodies and are the building blocks of our immunity. When our immune system is weak, we get sick easily. Hence, the words "immune compromised." So then, why is it that sometimes, you still become ill even when you sleep well, eat well, exercise, and drink your vitamins?

This could mean that the irritant or microorganism is too strong for your body to handle. It could have been attacking you, or you could have been exposed to it constantly for long periods of time. This is known as chronic exposure. Your soldiers are unable to hold them back or fight them any longer. It overcomes your soldiers, and you find yourself falling ill.

Our body have many layers of protection. Although the WBCs are not the only protection our body has, it proves that in normal circumstances it is not so easy for the body to become ill.

The body does not only contain the physical but also the energy body, which includes the mental and emotional aspects and the spiritual body. The physical body has, foremost, the skin, which already has two layers: the epidermis (skin surface) and dermis (just below the epidermis). Then there is the fat tissue, also known as adipose, located just below the epidermis. There's blood and blood vessels, along with the nervous system. We also have muscles, tendons, and joints. There are also bones, which maintain our physical structure. Then we have energy, also known as Qi, and the meridian channels, which are energy pathways where energy flows. You will find more information about Qi, energy, and meridian channels in many Traditional Chinese Medicine- or Oriental Healing Practices-related books. The energy and the meridian channels run throughout the body and are both directly and indirectly connected to your body's organs. Our organs include the heart, the brain, the lungs, liver, gallbladder, kidneys, stomach, and many others. After the organs, we also have the organ systems, which are interrelated to each other. Each system works with one another. For instance, your nose, which is part of the skin and your respiratory system, inhales air, which then goes to your lungs. Oxygen is then transported into the blood from the lungs to the heart. The heart pumps the blood through the blood vessels. The blood carries oxygen to all parts of the body to maintain viability. A viable stomach and digestive system aids in the breakdown and transformation of food. Food goes to the liver for metabolism then goes to the urinary system to be filtered and eliminate wastes. These are just some of the ways that show how they are related to one another.

The energetic body is what you sense and what you feel that is often, for most people, invisible to the naked eye. For some, they can see and feel energy such as seeing someone's aura.

Remember a time when you got a "boo-boo" when you were a child?—an injury from playing, whether a bruise, a scratch or a wound? With or without medication, your mother would place her loving hands around it, kiss it, and embrace you. Do you remember somehow feeling better? Although the pain may not have completely gone away, you felt better, and you felt warm, comfortable, and safe.

That is a form of energy. Similarly, when you feel down and someone offers you a listening ear, kind words, an open heart, and a hug, you suddenly feel a little bit better.

All living things are energy and carry energy. Your thoughts, your words, and your actions are all energy. Emotions and intentions are also forms of energy. Even certain areas or rooms have lingering energy. Think about stepping into a night club, a church, or a spa. The energy or the feeling is different in each location. You can sense this, which means you can sense energy.

Thoughts and words can heal or can hurt someone. There is power behind them. When you think, believe, and say, "I hate you! You are a stupid, good for nothing human being!," there is a negative and harmful energy that is being transmitted. When the receiving person cannot see or recognize this and is unable to manage these kinds of energies, they will not know how to protect themselves from such vibrational frequencies, thereby being affected by it. Taking on someone else's emotions and energy can be very confusing, as you might think it your own.

There was a time I was taking care of a patient who was very anxious, angry, and had cursed at me, knowing full well that how he felt about himself was being projected out to whoever happened to be around—which was me. I had been taking care of this patient almost all day long, being around him and helping him. Recalling back, the longer I took care of him, the more guarded and tense my whole body became. My shoulders started to rise up, tightening themselves; my brain became tense trying to keep the space in harmony; my whole chest and abdominal region tightened to keep my emotions in check and remain understanding but set boundaries as well. On top of that, this man was not my only patient. I also had to collaborate with many hospital staff. I was holding all of that in my body throughout most of the day.

Whenever you feel these physical changes happen in your body, before things get even more intense, it is important to remember to take a breath and exhale deeply. Allow the tension and tightness to be released each time you exhale. I remember coming home that day feeling not only exhausted but angry and anxious, although there was nothing to be angry or anxious about. That day pretty much ended, and I was just driving home. I should have been relaxed and looking forward to rest. Instead, I arrived home and out of nowhere, I took my frustration and anger out on my loved one. I thought to myself, "What's happening to you? What's your problem? Why are you like this? Why are you angry over a small nothing?" I realized that I had taken home someone else's energies that were not my own. I ended up apologizing, but it was already after I had hurt someone I loved. From then, I grew to learn to distinguish energies that were confusing to me. I'm still learning whether or not what I'm feeling is mine, or if it is someone else's. This is a practice I actively chose and intentionally cultivated in myself. From this experience, I decided that every day when I get home, I would make it a point to, before I enter the house, consciously assess what I'm feeling and visualize leaving behind the tensions of the day. I tell myself that anything less than love will not be allowed to enter in my home and that I need to practice this every day.

Whenever you interact with another human being, it is a good idea to also watch and be aware of yourself. Sometimes, you may notice a headache start to creep up when there was none in the beginning. Or perhaps you let out a big sigh of relief, releasing all the heaviness and tension you've been holding in your chest and shoulders being in the space you were just in. You may notice that you feel pain and discomfort in your body. You may be taking on someone else's burden or the situation itself is what is giving you these reactions in your body.

When you notice these signs and symptoms start to happen in your body, take time to focus on yourself and your breathing. Be aware of whether you are losing energy or losing a part of yourself in the situation. If you can, step away from the stressful environment you are in, even for just for a couple of minutes, and take some time to breathe, clear, and cleanse. Help release some, if not all, of the tension you are carrying.

The more we do not notice or regard these events or moments in our lives, no matter how small or big, and are unable to release what we have taken on as our own, the more these can get compounded on by the next similar interaction or situation. It can pile up to the point that our bodies may not be able to manage all of the burdens they are carrying, which can consequently predispose us to becoming ill.

It is also equally important to choose what words you use because they do not only affect the person you are talking to, they also affect your person. Being around yourself, the words you use and the thoughts you think can either bring you down, comfort you, or lift you up. It's up to you what words you will allow in your life. How you talk to others is really how you talk to yourself. I am not saying you cannot be angry, as anger can be productive, but think more on the choice of words you use when in a heightened emotion as much as you do in your everyday life.

Emotions are also energy and can be felt in the body. Emotions occur when there is a disruption in your flow or your way of life. They also come up when your desires, goals, or expectations are not fulfilled. It is like driving your car on a highway when suddenly someone from the next lane jumps in front of you abruptly without signaling. It jars you from your flow of driving. You can feel your emotions start to awaken, having thoughts of why you are angry or feeling incredulous. At the same time, your body starts to feel tense and tight. Your shoulder tenses, your chest and your abdominal muscles tighten, your whole body stresses out. We often do not notice or mind these things that our body go through in relation to our emotions. It is not that the situations create your emotions, it is actually you creating emotion from situations. Let me clarify. The car jumping in front of you does not carry emotion. It is what your body felt and perceived when it did that created the emotion. The emotion did not come from the car. It came from your body. That means emotions live in our body. It does not make us who we are. Instead, emotions are our tools to grow ourselves. They give us the space to be aware of our body and feelings.

In Traditional Chinese Medicine and Eastern Holistic Practices, certain emotions are related to the body's organs. Anger is connected to the liver. Joy is connected to the heart. Grief is to the lungs. Fear is to the kidneys. Worry is to the stomach and spleen. Do you notice that when you feel happy or in love, your heart feels warm and open? When people get extremely scared, they can easily lose urinary function and wet themselves. When you worry too much, your digestion is most likely not flowing well, and you might get diarrhea, constipation, acid reflux or feel bloated. When you are in extreme emotional pain, perhaps when someone very close to you just passed away, you may have difficulty breathing because your chest feels so tight from the sadness and pain of your loss. Being aware of the emotions that come up and the emotions that we create and how to manage them is also important in maintaining balance in our physical body.

Stress triggers our body, mind, and emotions. It is like a download or a virus that comes into the computer—the computer being us. It triggers the computer to respond. Stress can be healthy and can be used to our advantage to grow our body, our mind, and our spirit. However, prolonged exposure to stress and being unable to manage the stress creates imbalance. These imbalances can then manifest into physical symptoms if left unchecked.

There are many factors related to stress. These include the responsibilities we have, such as taking care of the family, especially our children, our work, paying bills to maintain our house and car, having adequate food and water, and many more. Relationships with other human beings can also create stressors, especially when we disagree with one another. In this case, we either let go what we feel or hold things in to prevent conflict with those we love or care about. Most often it is the latter. We tend to hold things in, and we might think that we have let them go, but instead, they can stay and live in your body, and if not processed well, may manifest into your physical body. Holding things in, suppressing our feelings, and being unable to express ourselves effectively and efficiently creates a disconnect within our mind, our body, and our spirit. It manifests and wreaks havoc in our body. Our body's response is actually an indicator of the imbalance between these three bodies, the mind, physical body, and the spirit.

When your body is under stress, it can be in a fight or flight response. Imagine you are out camping and a bear shows up hungry right outside your tent. How do you think your body is going to feel? Your heart rate could increase a little, if not a lot. Your breathing may quicken and become short and shallow. Your body is in high alert, tense, ready to fight or run. These reactions, whether large or small, when prolonged can create a significant impact on your physical body. Imagine being in this state for long periods of time—days, months, or for some, even years. How long do you think your body is going to handle all of this without taking a break?

You can watch how your body reacts under stress. When you know you are in this state, know that it is important to take a break. Take adequate time to reset and recover.

When you think of something that triggers the fires of anger in you although the situation has already passed, such as a divorce, a separation, or a cheating partner, you may think that you have let it go even though you still speak bitterly about it. You may think that it was so long ago that you should have been over it and done with already. If you feel even a slight judgement or emotional trigger about the circumstance, it only means that you have not completely processed it, and it still is stored in the back of your mind and your body is holding the space of your mind. Similarly, if you have grieved a loved one who passed away and their memory is still very painful even if it has been years, that means you still have grief. On the other hand, if the memory of your loved one creates a feeling of nostalgic celebration of joyous memories, you will sense a freedom and calm happiness.

Living on this earth as humans, we need to be provided with our basic needs—the things we need to survive. We need shelter, food, water. We need a safe space to live. These are basic necessities that need to be fulfilled. Without these, as humans, we will not survive in this physical world. There are many people who have gone through difficulties in their lives and have to work extra hard to survive. Many are able to get themselves out of poverty, hunger, and unsafe situations. They do all that they can with all that they have to support their families and each other until they pull themselves out of their situations and provide a better living for themselves and their families. Many have succeeded in this aspect. However, this can take a toll on the body and the psyche. On the other hand, they also grow in perseverance, strength, gratefulness, and compassion. Oftentimes, we do not focus on the positive that we took away from a situation but more on the negative or what is bad. We often disregard the good, and this is precisely why we need to acknowledge this growth in ourselves. Receive all the gifts you have been given and grown in yourself from the stressors and circumstances that you faced. These gifts are precisely what you need to help manage and navigate through your life in the present and in your future.

Actually, the earth has the capability to provide us with all that we need. It is the living conditions and the earth conditions that humans have created that cause some people to have this need unfulfilled. For most of the population on the planet, basic human needs are met. When this happens, we move on to material things: having a nice job, a nice car, a nice house in a nice neighborhood; having beautiful expensive clothes, bags, shoes, and accessories. These things can make us happy for a time.

We buy clothes, and we are happy; then the feeling goes away, and we buy again, and the cycle goes on. Material things, you will find, are not the basis of happiness. Money may make you happy for some time. It can help you live comfortably, but it does not define your happiness. I have a friend who knows someone who has a lot of money, multiple expensive cars, and lives in a beautiful mansion with a beautiful wife and children but is unable to sleep. Sleeplessness is affecting his life and making him miserable.

Would you rather have a lot of money, be unhappy, and be unable to sleep? Or is it better to have enough, be happy, and have peace of mind? What is most important to you? Surely, you can also have both plenty of money and be happy, right? It's all about balance. But money does not mean you will be happy. Money and material things do not define happiness. They do not guarantee peace of mind. They are tools to help you live comfortably.

I want to talk about money because it is also a form of energy. It is the value people place on a piece of paper. In reality, it is just a piece of paper with printing on it. It is the value we hold on it that we use to exchange services and materials. Money should serve to make your life easier and not be what makes your life hard. Let me repeat that:

"Money should serve to make your life easier, not make it difficult."

If this phrase is the opposite of what is happening in your life and you desire this saying to be the reality of your life, then you may want to reassess and readjust the way you are choosing to live your life.

Many people work so much and so hard, making little time for themselves, overworking until it affects their health to earn a lot of money to acquire material things or things that are non-basic or essential needs of survival. Sometimes I ask myself, "If I am not enjoying this, if my body is being affected by this, why am I killing myself over this? What is really important to me? Do I really need that expensive dress or jewelry? Is this three-bedroom house or high end luxury car really necessary for my happiness? Is this need more important than my health?" In other words, "Are you going to kill yourself over something you think you need to make your life comfortable?"

You could be thinking that this comfort is what is going to make you and your family happy. Are you going to kill yourself over that house, that dress, that car, that luxury life, that possible future, and is that what happiness means for you? In perspective, the question really is, "Are you going to kill yourself for what you think happiness might be?"

I am not saying you cannot get that expensive dress or jewelry you want or live in that three-bedroom house or own a luxury car. Of course, you absolutely can. I am talking about having a balance—a balance in taking care of yourself and your body. We put out so much of ourselves, so much energy and effort, and don't give ourselves enough time to recharge. Sometimes, there is a need to work overtime, many jobs, or be busy for the purpose of your own growth. But if you're in a situation where you want more money or to acquire material things but the process is detrimental to your health, a balance needs to happen. Reassess what is most important in your life. Figure out what happiness means for you. List what your main priorities are and number what your top three or five are in accordance with your heart. Your number one should be what makes you happy and what lights the fire of your spirit.

Believe that it will work out because you will work it out so long as you do not forget to take care of yourself. Again, an imbalance can lead to discomfort and dis-ease or unease of the body. It can certainly affect your physical health.

I recall working with this man named John. He came to me because he felt like he was in the right place in his life at that moment but something felt disconnected that he could not figure out. This had been bothering him and affecting his life. He had been hopping from one job to another, not really putting much importance or effort into the responsibilities of the work itself, much like a sense of loss of direction. John had just found a new job, and he had many good friends whom he had a great relationship with.

Everything that came up for the first thirty minutes of our session were all relevant to his life, but I did not feel that they were the reasons that were causing him confusion and disconnect. I also felt that he needed the space to gather the courage to really get to the root cause of things. Everyone is different in their process and for John, he needed the space to get himself comfortable first. It is a space that needed to be filtered. It was when he talked about a friend, being very subtle about it, that I saw the deep connection and spark in his being. I had to really catch that, backtrack, and bring that to light. He was having conflicting feelings about his really good friend, Suzy, because he started to fall in love with her. Suzy was in a relationship with someone else and often confided in John whenever she had trouble with her boyfriend. John tried to disregard or avoid this feeling that was growing, but it was something that needed to be acknowledged, as it was affecting his life and thought processes. This was really the most significant thing in his life that impacted his living—not the stressors of the responsibilities of the new job or the previous jobs. I helped John realize that he was in a habit of trying to make everyone comfortable around him and not giving his truth importance. He always felt the need to ease people into receiving and accepting his message and ultimately really accepting who he was as a person. I helped him realize that it was not necessary to waste a lot of time, energy, and effort trying to please people to make them like or accept who he was, especially when they were supposed to be his friends. He wanted to be that good friend, good person, so it conflicted with his growing feelings for Suzy. This caused bouts of energy as well as moments of worrying, overthinking, and fatigue throughout the day. I sensed that this was the disconnect the body was manifesting in physical form. His energy and focus were also scattered, which was a reflection of his life.

John was finally able to focus on what Suzy's significance was to him and his life. I helped shine a light on what his heart truly desired. Would he be absolutely okay with whatever outcome resulted from his decision, whatever it may be? Was that really what his heart was telling him? I helped him free the clutter in his mind to clear out the confusion it was causing. He needed to bring about his courage to find the truth about what the meaning of happiness is for him. Being clear and honest with yourself and what your heart wants is important so you can choose to align your decisions with your truth. Pretending or trying so hard to make others like you or accept you can cause extreme stress and ultimately can be very exhausting. We do not realize that it takes so much effort to hide our true selves just so we feel like we belong. It can be a source of fatigue from hidden and buried sadness.

Sometimes, it is important to stop and pause, especially when you are confused, to really think about what makes you happy. When you have your answer, ask yourself, "Are you sure that that is your answer, or is there really something else you do not want to face because of fear of losing what you already have right now? What you have right now is comfortable and safe, but does it make you happy?" Most often when faced with this question stemming from deep inside you, the answer is NO. Why are you in a state of confusion when you are unhappy and unsatisfied with how things are in your life right now?

You might say, "I have everything I could possibly need and want in my life, so why do I feel like it is not enough? I should be grateful, and I am, but why does it feel like something is missing? Why does this not make me happy anymore when it had made me happy in the past?" Do not fret when you don't get your answer right away. It is a start in knocking on the door of deep truth that you have so guarded and protected so strongly. It is a great thing. Finding what true happiness is for you is a wonderful revelation. It may not seem like it when you are going through this phase, but I am telling you that it is a great and beautiful thing. When you see someone who is bright and vibrant, full of life, admired by many for being courageous, gracious, and inspirational, living their truth, and sharing their authentic self, you will find that as you get to know them, you will know that they went through their nitty gritty rock-polishing phase too. So I say, do not be afraid! You are not alone in finding that balance, finding that happiness, hope, and peace within yourself. I feel that our physical body is a great indicator, messenger, and motivator in helping us get to that space. So I say, "Thank you, my body, for showing me what I need to work on. I am truly humbled and grateful."

"The first wealth is health!
–Ralph Waldo Emerson

This saying, to me, means that if you have your health, there are infinite possibilities. If you are healthy, you can go for what you want, get what you need, and pursue your heart's desires. You can still do the same even if you are not healthy, but it will be a lot harder. If you are healthy, you can work, make money, and be more effective in being of service. If you are sick, you stay home, feel miserable, are unable to work, and it makes it more difficult for you to achieve your goals.

Being ill does not mean it is the end of your world. A lot of times, it simply means an imbalance in your body—a disconnect between your body, your mind, and your spirit. Many times, it is your body signaling you that something is wrong; you need to look into it, take a rest, or take care of yourself. It could also mean that the body is now at war with whatever imbalance, irritant, or foreign bodies are trying to attack it. You need to find a space of support for your body to recover. This is why we eat well, drink plenty of water, and get lots of sleep when we get sick. We create a supportive environment for our body to fight and bring our body back to homeostasis or a normal state.

Imbalance of the body can also mean that it is at war, a disconnect between your thoughts, your heart, your actions, and your words. How we present or express ourselves to others may not be what we truly want or mean. We tend to do this when we do not want to hurt another person or we just want to get along and go along with what the majority wants or expects, not knowing that we are hurting ourselves. When we are not in alignment with our truth, our spirit is not happy. We feel we cannot truly show or be who we are. Your physical body actually feels this. Do you remember the emotions that wash over you when you are hiding something or not telling the whole truth? How did your body react and how uncomfortable did your body feel? Is this how you really want to be? I say it is better not to say anything when it is meant to hurt or destroy and when your opinions and words will harm someone. Speaking your truth, even when it hurts, for the purpose of growth and healing is necessary and is a great thing. Lessons of life are not always dainty and nice, flowers and diamonds. It can be a hard-core, nitty gritty stubborn rock that has to go through grease and mud, go through miles of turbulent rapids of life, as you already well know. This piece of rock can be polished into a diamond to shine bright in this world and create happiness not only for yourself but for others as well if you allow it to. This is why it is equally important to find the time and space to clear out the cobwebs and be clear in your connection to your heart and your spirit as much as creating a space for your physical body to recover, reset, and rejuvenate to homeostasis. They are not separate, as resting your physical body is also a rest and breathing room for your mind, body, and spirit.

Stress can also bring about worry and anxiety. Worry and anxiety stem from not knowing what's going to happen or what the outcome is. It comes from not being in control of the results. We often worry about things that are out of our hands. That is because we are not open to the disruption of the flow in our life. We want it the way it is. I feel that when I worry about something not in my control, my head gets fuzzy and tight, and my stomach or abdominal region become cold and feel uneasy. I feel I am holding my breath, and my body is tense. Prolonged worrying eventually brings about the onset of persistent gnawing headache or migraine. It is my brain saying, "This is too much for me! I am in so much stress/pain that I cannot and do not want to think about anything right now. I need a break!" Even so, we often neglect this message. Many thoughts coursing through your head can get your head overheated. Replaying what happened, what could have happened, if only this, if only that, can be used for growth, but when you constantly replay things in your mind like a broken record, then it becomes unhealthy. It can affect your physical body.

I used to be in a habit of worrying too much. Along the way of my life, I became a worrier. I figured out that worrying too much was my habit and worked to cope differently. If something is beyond my control, I do not need to spend my energy on something that isn't there. I realized that I was constantly creating scenarios of possible outcomes or results that may or may not even happen. I was creating stories that were not necessary. I was unaware that doing this gave me shoulder pains, a heavy feeling of the head, migraine headaches, and a poor quality of sleep. Thoughts continued running in my head nonstop and when I slept, sometimes I got disconcerting dreams. I woke up feeling exhausted and spent. This is because I was fully mentally awake when I was supposed to be sleeping, at rest, or in a relaxed state. A relaxed state promotes rejuvenation, repair, and balancing of the body. In addition, this worrisome attitude also made me have very little appetite, feel bloated, and feel like I was unable to digest food well. I felt like my metabolism slowed down. I was gaining weight even with little sleep, little eating, and lots of stress. I only realized this correlation between my thoughts and physical symptoms as I became aware of my own habits and emotions when I decided to start listening to my body. I saw how my physical symptoms were actually messages signaling me that something was not right. There was an imbalance that needed to be addressed and taken care of.

When it comes to worrying and overthinking, I have learned to trust that if there is nothing I can do, if something is beyond my hands or my power, then whatever is meant to happen is going to happen. I remind myself that it takes practice to change a habit. It does not take overnight to change the part of me that I made as my own. I decided that whatever the result will be, I will face it when I cross that bridge.

In the meantime, I use the energy I would use for this unnecessary worrying for something else worthwhile. Worry takes a lot of time and effort. It is an unnecessary effort. It affects not only your digestion and your heart but also your peace of mind.

I remember a time that my head became too hot and heavy, even when I didn't have a fever. I was having a really bad headache from overthinking and over-worrying, and it was difficult for me to take a break from my own running thoughts. I was exhausted and could not fully rest. I said to myself, "What can I do that will help me quickly slow down my thoughts? I need to cool my head and just pause from thinking. My brain is working too hard and needs a break." I decided to fill the sink with cold water and submerge my head in the water. I could almost feel the sizzle from my hot head in contrast to the cold water as I put my head under. I focused on the feel and solitude of the water, devoid of unnecessary chatter. It was quite refreshing and helped me slow down my thoughts. I noticed it was helping, so I repeated it a few times until my head started to feel better. Knowing the principle of energetic balance of the body, I also put a warm pack on my belly and just lay down on the bed. I realized that I was losing energy and losing power from my core because it was being used by my brain and unnecessary thoughts. My abdomen had felt clammy, bloated, and empty. I focused on the warmth of my abdomen, and I felt my body become comfortable enough that I consequently fell asleep. I had a really restful sleep that time and woke up feeling refreshed and ready for the new day.

Sometimes it is exercise that helps me clear my head and open up my body. Sometimes it is sleep that help me recover more that the exercise. Each person and each situation can be different in how to reset and recover. This is why it is essential to know your own body and know what works best in whatever situation you are in that warrants clearing and cleansing.

When we have our basic needs met, money and material things included, we next often look for success and recognition. We want to be recognized for our achievements. This is why we work extra hard to be acknowledged. We desire our existence to be recognized. This is why you work hard to get awards, to be known, to have a lot of money to get that fancy car, get that beautiful house in that high end neighborhood, get those brand name dresses and luxury bags. If you want to be recognized just to feel good, then that is just your Ego talking. But, if your purpose is to be recognized and be successful to be of service to many others, then that is different. That is your spirit talking. They say success comes with great responsibility. You can see why true success does not serve your Ego and does not equal happiness. You can have everything you need and every material thing you want but feel it is never enough. Even with recognition, your Ego will never be satisfied. It is only with great humbling responsibility that success works. So unless the spirit is at work, you will always be running *after* success and recognition. If your spirit or soul is at work, then you will be running *in* the embrace of success and recognition. When you allow your soul to shine through, success and recognition are the extras that come along with it. When we have our basic needs met and we have enjoyed the fruits of our labor, some might then get to the level of, what next? What now? You might feel stuck. When you find yourself in this space, it is important to also know about your spirit body because the connection with your heart, mind, and spirit will help you find your answer.

The spiritual body is connected to our heart and mind. Having a healthy and strong relationship between your heart and your mind allows your soul to shine through. Our spiritual body is currently housed in our physical body for the time being until our physical body passes away. So this is why it is important to also take good care of your physical body.

All parts and all aspects of our body are important. They are related to each other, which means one can easily affect the other. This indicates that each one can also help the other. My definition of optimal well-being is having a clear and healthy connection between your heart, your mind, and your spirit along with your physical body. So it is extremely important to be mindful and aware of all aspects of our body: the physical body, energy body and spiritual body—the body, mind, and spirit connection.

What I've mentioned thus far are many of the things that clutter our mind and weaken our body. Clearing the mind and cleansing the body helps you set a base for your healing, like the preparation and the washing of the ingredients in baking or cooking.

In the same way, we need to prepare what is necessary and wash away the dirt and clutter that is not needed to clear and cleanse the mind and the body for healing.

Clearing the mind means emptying your thoughts and having a feeling of neutrality. That means that there is absolutely no noise, ideas, words, or thoughts that are running in your mind. It feels like the wind passing through air and just letting your brain breathe. When you come to a state of zero thoughts, you will feel neutrality. No thoughts equals no emotions. Our thoughts generate our emotion and whatever emotion comes up, our physical body responds to it.

Thoughts and emotions are normal parts of life. They are necessary for our growth. However, chronic and persistent unhealthy thoughts and emotions can create imbalances in our health. If our body is unable to sustain this prolonged imbalance, it could very well become something permanent and can create disease. Each individual has their own capabilities and level of healing depending on their relationship with the aspects of their bodies. This is why it is important to give our mind and body a breather when it desperately needs it.

Rest and reset equals clearing the mind and cleansing the body.

There are many ways to achieve clearing and cleansing. Exercise, stretching, meditation, spa, massage, tub baths, martial arts, aromatherapy, acupuncture, running, dancing, walking in the park, sitting on the sand beach, being around nature and breathing in its beauty, and even sleeping are some of the many ways that you can help clear your head and cleanse the mind.

There are days that you need the sleep more than the exercise.

There are days that you need the massage more than the running.

The more you learn and are connected to your body, your mind, your thoughts and emotions, the more you will know what works for you and what helps you.

Spending time in nature is a great way to help detox the mind and help relax the body. Breathe in the fresh air, listen to the birds and the wind, watch the trees sway, feel the breeze against your cheek. If you are at the beach, you can relax by the water, put your feet in the sand, and feel yourself connected to the earth, listen to the waves, and look out into the horizon of the sky and just breathe. Let everything go. Let everything out. Nothing else matters except that moment.

Exercise can also help you clear your mind by enabling you to focus on one task that is challenging. It helps strengthen your body, your mind, and your spirit. Stretching your body, you will realize, is also stretching your mind. Your body makes you feel and see your mind as you stretch or as you run or exercise. It is your spirit and your mind that tells you and wills you to choose to stretch your body or go exercise because it is what you need. This is an example of how the mind, the body, and the spirit are all connected.

Breathing is important because it is life. Without breath, our physical body will not survive. We often take for granted the joy and gift of breathing. Being aware of your breath and how it enters and exits your body effectively and positively is another way to help cleanse the body. You can sit comfortably and watch your breath come into your lungs or chest and come out through your mouth. See how your body is reacting to your breathing.

Release the tension in your brain, your shoulders, and your body as you breathe out. When your body relaxes, your mind also relaxes. If you ever had the best massage of your life before, do you remember the feeling your body and your mind felt? After the massage, I remember having zero thoughts and just feeling good.

My brain could breathe, and my body was warm and comfortable.

My body had released tension, and my mind was empty and clear.

I felt like a fresh start.

Meditation is also a great way to help you be clear about your life. It can give you a space of safety to be able to hear and connect with your heart and spirit. It can be a haven to feel your soul.

A clear mind and a warm body are the base you want for your healing. Strengthening your core or your abdominal region helps strengthen your body. Being aware of your breathing can help open up your chest and warm your heart. Having a cool head helps clear the mind. This is the flow you want to be in, the flow to reset your body and your mind.

It is important to have a conversation and a connection with your body. The more you tune in, the more you will learn what your body needs and when it needs help. You will learn what works for you and what doesn't. The next step will share about going in depth in this process.

Chapter 6
STEP 2—Listen and Feel

T ake a minute to close your eyes and watch your breath. Listen to the sound of your breathing. Think of nothing and feel your chest. This may be easier said than done. Just try and keep practicing. When you are learning something new, it is often normal to not get it right away. It takes practice and effort. So do just give it a try and see how you feel.

Close your eyes and watch your breath. Your breath is the most important thing in your life at this moment. Nothing else matters. Breathing is essential in continuing to live in the physical world. Watch your body as you inhale, watch and let your chest expand, only thinking of your breathing. Watch as your body exhales, letting out as much air as you can from your lungs and watch how your body responds. Go ahead and give it a try. Set the alarm and just do this for two minutes.

What did you feel? Was that not the longest two minutes you have experienced? Your body can be like the ocean when you learn how to utilize it. I say this because, just like sitting by the beach, listening to the waves and the wind, breathing fresh air, you can do the same with your own body. Like the beach can melt your stresses away even for a moment, you can practice doing the same with your own body.

The body has the capacity to tell you what feels good and what does not. Your stomach tells you if something is bad or if something feels healthy. Your nose tells you if something smells good or smells funky. Your body provides you with many messages.

When you overdo a workout, your body feels aches and pains, screaming, "This is too much. Get some rest!" If you have not moved your body for a long time and started exercising in moderation, your pain might be telling you, "It's about time you started moving me. I was getting stagnant and do not want to waste away. This pain feels good." You will learn the difference between the body screaming at you as opposed to the body saying, "Ah, I can finally move, breathe and stretch. Thank you! Finally!" You will know what healing pain feels like versus screaming pain. Learning to listen to your body's messages is a start to a close and special relationship with yourself.

Growth and healing need time to process. However long or short the time is depends on the person. When I broke up with my former fiancé, I was in a lot of hurt and was depressed. I cried every time I woke up and any time there were gaps of emptiness during the day. I watched many TV series and made myself busy. Work helped me keep my mind off of the pain. That same year, I learned about energetic healing. I found that I had a preconception about the time it takes to heal from a heartbreak. I thought it was going to take a long time, perhaps two years, to move on.

Surprisingly, throughout the process of healing, I focused on myself and had a candid conversation with my truth. This helped me process very quickly. I am able to remember the whole breakup, but I knew for sure what I needed, what I truly wanted, and what felt right and pure to me. I realized how my perception of pain was an illusion that I made so much bigger than what it was. I saw with clarity that the love I have inside is so much more abundant than the speck of pain I was spreading all over myself. From then, I realized that healing takes place depending on how honest you can be with yourself and how ready you are to face yourself.

I was not brought up in a society that considers opening up yourself as the norm. Trying to show that you are strong, that the vulnerable can depend on you, and showing that you can handle the situation are what was expected even though deep down, you were also struggling and hurting. This is pretend strength. Real strength comes from being honest with yourself and others. This realness and this true strength need to be nurtured.

It was a widespread belief in the past that parents, older siblings, and men in general are supposed to be the rock or the strength. Also, if you have been a fighter all your life, fighting for survival or fighting to prove others wrong, this is most likely your normal defense mechanism as well. You might have tried to hold your tears, hold your emotions in check, especially when others are around. This suppression does not let the flow of the process go through. In time, it becomes stagnant and creates tightness in the chest, shortness of breath, or difficulty speaking your truth, feeling a lump in your throat. You are unable to express yourself well with pent up emotions.

Crying is a form of release, as is communicating what matters or what bothers you. Things can become stuck if suppressed. These can be carried in our body if not processed well. In the long run, this could possibly manifest in something tangible. When you need to cry, take time to fully commit in your grieving. Do not cut short your expression of release. Invite the pain to fully process through. Watch your body as your chest and lungs are being squeezed. Let go of what burdens your heart. Once you have fully let yourself be free and allowed yourself to be vulnerable, you will feel a sense of relief and release from your chest. That squeeze you felt before can transform into a breath of clarity and freshness. This was my experience when my aunt, who was like a mother to me, suddenly passed away. I welcomed and fully embraced all the pain and grief that I was feeling. I knew that it was the way to move forward and grow into healing.

There was a time when I was working in the Surgical Intensive Care Unit as a nurse that I had a lot of stresses and was angry that I could not articulately explain myself the way I wanted and often felt misunderstood. At the time, I was sporadically teaching yoga classes as well and going on trainings to improve myself. I knew that my body was holding a lot due to the stress. Although it was busy and I was moving around physically and constantly, my body felt very tight and stiff by the time I got off work. Knowing this, I would train to release my tensions and what I was holding in every time I got off work. I remember a week that was extremely heavy. By the third day of work, as I was getting deeper in my release training, I felt a tangible lump on my liver area that had never been there before. It just showed up out of nowhere. Keeping in mind that I had been doing trainings the past two days, I had not noticed a lump there before. There was a certain type of feeling and energetic frequency that I knew was not normal. It was a tension my body had formed. The first thing that came to mind was, "Oh my gosh! This is how cancer starts!" Intuitively, that was my first thought.

To explain it differently, this is akin to having to move your bowels but holding it in for a long time, unable to pass it. It gets compacted, hard, and your abdomen starts to become hard and firm, now unable to expel it or release it and later on can cause infection. You may need to take many medications, and if unresolved, it may cause complications and you may end up needing surgery.

In my case, it was my liver area. I hardly drink alcohol, and I do not eat too many fatty or oily foods, but it was there. It alarmed me a little, but I knew exactly what I needed to do. It took me two hours that day to release that tension alone. I had my yearly check up with the doctor, and everything was normal.

How much more does our body need to endure and struggle when we are not aware of it and its messages? We can easily get into the habit of carrying this tension around thinking that this is the norm. It can become the body's natural state when it really is unnatural. Some people do not even realize that they are walking around with a headache, a stiff neck, or tense shoulders. It is harder to distinguish that a heavy head is actually a form of headache because your body believes it to be in a natural state. You only find out that it is a headache once it is released. When this occurs, it is much more challenging to get the body to recognize homeostasis, the normal state. Even after getting the body soft and relaxed, the body reverts back to what it believes to be the norm, which is a tension state. So although it may take some time, extra effort is needed for the body to recognize what is the natural state it needs to be in.

It is important to distinguish between what is natural and what is not. It is equally essential to also know the difference between your truth and a misconception. I had been working with a woman named Lorna who had been absolutely unhappy with her life for some time. She was constantly exhausted and felt drained every day. She slept enough hours and ate appropriately but continued to feel fatigue all the time. She just moved out from a rural area in England and into London. She took on a job with a higher pay and opted to not spend as much time with her friends. Lorna felt that she was not being a good friend, as she felt that she should be in a better position because she was more senior and an older employee. Her younger friends got the upgrades or the promotions, and she felt left behind. She saw her friends happy, and she felt guilty that she felt envious.

As a true friend, she should be happy for them and not feel jealous, wanting to have what they had. Initially, the sadness might have easily been mistaken for her long distance relationship with her husband and family and being away from them. But it was actually about how she felt about herself. Lorna had been living with guilt and shame for being a horrible friend and human being. She always aimed to be a good person and try to be honest with her feelings. This time, she could not help but feel this way. Lorna had isolated herself from her friends and focused her time and energy on work. Sifting through the energetic barriers and listening in to what her heart was really saying, I helped her realize that what she really wanted was to find her happiness. I asked Lorna, "Will you be happy if you have that position that your friends have? Do you think that being in that position will make you happy?" I knew the answer before she even replied, "No." She did not care so much about the promoted positions her friends got. Lorna knew deep down that it was not the upgrade or the position she really wanted but that she just needed to see that for herself. She had thought that if she got what her friends have, then she would be happy like her friends were. I helped her see that her friends' happiness was not necessarily her own. There was this misconception of being envious and being uncomfortable around her friends for not being true to herself, but in reality, it was actually the happiness she saw in her friends that she wanted to find for herself.

Desiring happiness for yourself does not make you a horrible friend or a terrible person. Knowing this is a start to truly listening to what you want and what your heart is saying. Feeling exhausted constantly for what seems to be no reason can be a cry to wake up. It can be a call to listen and feel your heart.

Whenever you feel chronic exhaustion but cannot figure out why, it is time to listen in. After clearing and cleansing, take time to be with yourself, have a sincere conversation, and really listen to yourself. You may often see within yourself the things that you do not want to face. You preoccupy yourself by being busy or doing other things to distract your mind from asking serious questions or looking deeper. There could be underlying reasons as to why you are feeling exhausted. Most often, I notice that it is primarily because you may not like your present reality anymore. You may have reveled in it in the past, but it does not do anything for your spirit anymore. I notice that many times chronic, unexplained exhaustion and tiredness is the dimming of a person's energy and spirit, the stepping back of the real self. It can be exhausting living a life that does not align with your passion and your truth. You may slowly be giving up on yourself and just trying to get by on what is expected of you and what you expect from yourself. Just getting closer, knowing the ins and outs of yourself, can shed light on what is the root issue of why you are feeling the way are feeling. You may find the answer to the question of, "Despite everything I have and I have all that I need, why does it feel like something isn't right with me?;" the answer to, "What's the matter with me when I have everything I could possibly want and need?;" the answer to, "What's wrong with me when everything seems to be fine?"

A society or a movement of acceptance and love need to shift in the mindset of humans. We are really not separate from each other. Just as Lorna has her story and I have my own, I'm sure you do too. You have your own story, your own struggles, your own heartaches that someone else is also going through, even if not necessarily exactly the same as you. We should not be quick to judge others no matter what the circumstances are. We go through our own life with all kinds of lessons just like others are doing the same. Pointing a finger at others and saying things you do not like about them is an indication that you need to look inward as well. Why am I so affected and impacted by this person or their actions? Is this something my heart is called to listen to and take action? Or is this a lesson of walking away from unnecessary distractions? Listen and feel yourself. Listen to your heart and feel your body. They are not separate.

Everything we go through in life, everyone we meet, and the environment we are exposed to all contribute to our health and well-being. So do not think that you are separate at all. But in order to hear others' calls for help, we need to answer our own call for help first. It is important to understand yourself in order to understand others.

As you become closer to all aspects of your body, you will learn when you need to conserve energy, when to share or circulate energy, and when you are losing your power. You will learn what you need to focus on and what you need to let go. You will know what challenges you need to tackle and which ones to walk away from.

Did you know that your stomach can also be related to your headaches? In my experience, oftentimes it's the blockages or stiffness of the shoulders, neck, or back that cause headaches. However, there was a time that I was working on releasing tension from my abdominal region when I hit a specific point by my stomach area. Whenever this point was stimulated, it caused a relief from my tension headache. At the time, due to a car accident I had, I couldn't really dance my heart out, which is usually one of the ways I clear and cleanse, so I did the belly button healing instead. The New York Times bestselling author Ilchi Lee talks about this method in his book, *I've Decided To Live 120 Years.* I rhythmically made movements in and out, engaging my belly button as I focused on my breathing. Medically, I have no digestive problems. This time I knew where my headache was coming from. It was from stress, overthinking, and worrying, which were related to the stomach.

Additionally, there was also a time when I had a headache surrounding my temples and on the top of my head. I thought, like before, it was coming from my stomach, but later on after doing some stretching, I learned that it was coming from my lower back instead, where my kidneys are located. I know I mentioned that the kidney is related to fear, but it is also related to overwork and fatigue. Oftentimes, when you do not get enough sleep and are working too much, this area gets tight and tense. My headache was telling me that I was overdoing things and that I had not been taking good care of myself like I should. Stretching and releasing the tension actually gave me relief from my headache. It helped even more after my beauty sleep. Without medication, my headache disappeared. I thought I knew where my headache was coming from, but I realized that I really need to pay more attention and be clear about the origin and meaning of my pain. Assuming it came from the same reason may be misleading. It is really important to have a connection and relationship with your body and truly listen and feel the messages your whole being is conveying.

When you get headaches that persist, not knowing where they are coming from, and when you have eliminated all the physical and medical factors that could be the cause, it is time to look within. Feel in your body where your symptoms are coming from and truly listen. Give your body the space to talk with you and really hear.

It is amazing to get to know your own body. It is empowering to know that although the doctor can help me, I can also really be at the forefront in helping myself.

I know that as I get older, my body is not as young and not as resilient as before, which is the more reason I should take better care of myself. All the more reason I need to have a close, intimate relationship with all aspects of myself.

In choosing to have a sincere relationship with yourself, you will often encounter the Ego. The Ego, growing up, was a form of security so you did not get hurt. It is, in a way, our defense mechanism. But as you get stronger, you should not let your security guard, "the Ego," be the leader of your life. Let Ego be the security when it needs to be, and let your true spirit be the master of your life.

Ego says, "It's my way or the highway. It has to be my way because my way is the best and only way." This stubbornness in siding with the Ego can create conflict, confrontations, and disharmony. It is the one who refuses to say sorry even when you are in the wrong or says sorry but with so much indignation and insincerity that it cancels out the apology. Being dishonest while holding a grudge holds a very heavy type of energy. It is confusing and can be very destructive to both you and the one you're aiming at.

Grudges are a form of suppression. You are holding in your feelings because you are hurt or embarrassed. You need to have a chat with yourself about whether or not this is helping you. Your Ego will want to hold on to it and exact revenge. On the other hand, your spirit will tell you that this is not helpful for you and that you should let it go. Believe that you are supported, especially when you choose to heal and grow yourself. Let go of what harms. Nurture what heals. Choose to be light and bright.

Most times, Ego shows up when we try to hide our insecurities. We want to prove that we are strong and that we can do it on our own, so we put up the wall of Ego so we do not become vulnerable and get hurt, made fun of, or taken advantage of. We hide our true self, our radiant self, behind the so-called tough guy, the Ego, just so to avoid being hurt.

Also, be aware that the feeling of being needed can also be a form of Ego. The Ego wants to be needed to feel good about themselves. "Look, I'm a good person because I am helping someone else. They need me and I am here." Know that when you do something for someone because it makes you feel good about yourself, it is not necessarily real love when you expect them to thank you, feel good about you, or like you. There is a fine line. Doing something in order to be needed, to be accepted, and be loved is the work of Ego. It is when you help and share yourself without expecting anything in return is when the spirit is at work. That is true giving.

Learn to receive criticism with grace. Again, you have the choice to either accept it or not accept it as your truth. Someone may say that the ocean is green, and someone might say it is red. You can choose to accept green, or red, or even none of the two. Sometimes, feedback is helpful so use it to your advantage. Other times, it is not, so you do not have to accept it as your truth.

It is your choice. Sounds simple, right? Wrong! For most people, it is not easy to accept criticism, especially when it hurts the Ego. It sounds simple, but putting it into action can be challenging especially when it is something you want to learn for yourself. Being aware of this will help you face your Ego without looking away. Just keep going and the more you choose your truth, the more your spirit will become stronger and brighter.

I know it is not as easy as it sounds. It is when your Ego faces another person's Ego that creates a huge divide. It is like a wall trying to ram itself into another wall. They force themselves on each other, and no one wants to give in or listen to the other with an open mind and an open heart. Each one wants to prove that they are right and that they are better than the other. The Ego wants to win to feel good about itself, despite knowing deep down that it can hurt the other. The Egos compete with each other while unconsciously disregarding the principle of choosing the universal good.

I remember clearly the first of many times I faced my Ego head on. It was during my vision quest. I was in a cave in Sedona, Arizona at the time when Ego was naturally being brought to the forefront. I had no say and had no control over my Ego. It just did its own thing in front of my eyes because I realized that I allowed it to run unchecked. It became a habit. I acknowledged that it was there, faced it squarely, swimming in my own discomfort and embarrassment. I was mortified knowing what I was doing but unable to stop my Ego from making a fool of myself. I saw it unfold in front of me and I could not make it stop going on and on. My Ego was talking and talking, justifying and rationalizing, making itself look great and mighty. Like a know it all, Ego stepped up and reared its head, rolling out defense mechanisms one after another. It was like an out-of-body experience where you become this separate entity, seeing yourself make a fool of yourself but unable to stop it. It was horrifying just to watch, but I watched myself through it all. I watched all kinds of emotions, pushing and pulling, fighting within and circulating all over my body. It was quite a long night in that cave. Fortunately, I was with people who are understanding, loving, and accepting because we were all supporting each other's growth. The next day, I acknowledged my Ego and spoke openly about it. Recognizing my own Ego and letting it know that I knew it was there but from now on, I was in charge and not Ego.

It is when we are disconnected from our truth and our spirit, being directed by our Ego and defense mechanisms, that we cannot truly show our true self. This creates a lot of discomfort in our physical body. If we choose to continue this path of disconnect, the body's unease and discomfort can become worse.

In time, through many more practices with my Ego and many more embarrassments, I learned to catch it when Ego wants to hijack my life. It is a work in progress. I learned to receive criticism and feedback more openly. Moreover, I learned to recognize others' Egos as well. I openly embrace them because I understand them. I choose to meet openly with my soul so their souls will recognize that I am choosing to interact with their truth and not the Ego. It is like knocking on a friend's door looking for your friend Rachel. Rachel's bodyguard, Evan the Ego, answers scowling, telling you to go away. Evan tries to push you away from Rachel because he does not want Rachel to get hurt in case you hurt her. You clearly see Evan's intention but decide to call and wait for Rachel to show up anyway. Rachel will eventually come out to meet you.

Rachel is the symbol of the truth, the authentic spirit, and the true master of the house. Evan the Ego is just working for Rachel. So Rachel needs to step up and be the Master, not Evan.

Of course, I still meet with my Ego time and again and still get to bump heads. I embrace it, my Ego, because it is a part of me. I am grateful for it to be my support and protector when I needed and helped me grow to be strong. But now, I need to step up and let my soul be the Master of my own life. The Master is all grown up and needs to lead the household.

I have faced my Ego countless times since I decided on the path of growth and healing, and I used to dread facing it, but I always look on the other side of it and see how much I have grown when I choose my spirit to be in charge. So now, I welcome whatever comes, even if it makes me vulnerable, embarrassed, or hurt because I know I will come out of it wiser and stronger. It is only my Ego that gets hurt, but my heart and soul grow. This, I felt, was all worth it. A transformation happens in the whole dynamic of a situation. A misunderstanding turns to a loving closeness. I've seen it happen many times. The disharmony melts away and changes into sincerity and respect. This may not always happen, but I have seen this transformation many times.

Facing your Ego is a part of your healing when you choose this path, so be prepared for it. Be prepared in feeling vulnerable, sensitive, hurt, and even embarrassed. The more you are faced with this, the more you will recognize Ego, and you will get to have a clear choice on who you choose to lead your life.

Chapter 7
STEP 3—Establish Action or Inaction

here is a saying in the Bible, "Ask and it shall be given unto you." This may be the case, but if you do not do your part, it will not come to fruition. For instance, you may ask to have a good job with good pay, but you never apply for any job. Jobs are available and are advertised on the newspaper, which you read every day. You pray to have a good job, but you do not take action in getting one.

Taking action creates movement of energy. The flow does not become stagnant, and there is room for growth and room for opportunities through changes. It creates a different circumstance or a change from what is already going on in your life.

Taking a leap into the unknown can be a scary thing. If you are unhappy and in pain, struggling to live your life, then what is stopping you from creating a change? What will fear do to you when you decide to take action? If anything, it will go away. You may create another fear or worry from the action you just took, but the original fear you have will disappear because you already changed the circumstance.

Change is what is constant. Everything is ever-changing and ever-moving. That is the flow of life. When you hold off or block the flow of life, it creates resistance to what is natural.

Acting on your decisions can inversely and directly affect not only yourself but those around you. Know who decided on taking action. The spirit is the one deciding when it is for the good of all and not for just one or the other but for universal wellness.

When it is just from pure selfish benefit, then it is from the limiting Ego. Align your action with your truth, and you can live without regret.

Effort is needed to create change. Practice and exercise action until it becomes a natural part of you. Make it second nature to develop your character as you take action in healing and growing yourself.

When a baby starts to stand and walk, the baby tries countless times, falling and getting up again, never giving up, until the baby is able to stand and walk on his/her own. Later on, walking and standing becomes second nature and without much effort or thought, they are easily done. We should do the same in developing our character. Practice who you want to be, who you are meant to be. You have the power to create the life that you want. Through practice and effort, it can become natural to you. Eventually, you will live how you want to be effortlessly.

Many times, we do not like change and choose to not take further steps because of fear. The fear of failure and the fear of the unknown stops us from moving forward. We are so used to what we know that we are afraid to step out of our comfort zone even when it is necessary. We wait until it becomes life or death or when we become sick to make a decision and take action.

"People want to change but they are afraid to actually make the change."

You desperately want to change your circumstance, but you are too afraid that things will change and it'll be a change that you may not like. You're afraid of what might or might not happen. It is like cutting your hair short when you only know and identify your hair to be long, your hair length reaching your mid-lower back. You've been used to and love having your hair long. It is a part of you that identifies you as a woman. But this time, it is summer, and you feel like you want a dramatic change. You are turning fifty years old, and you want your life to be simple and low maintenance. You feel like you simply have no time and patience for it anymore. You feel like your fifty should be the new thirty. You know full well that your hair will not grow as quickly or the same as it did when you were in your twenties. You feel the courage, fear, and excitement as you sit on the salon chair. When asked by the hairdresser, "How short do you want it to be?" he shows you your long hair, and what do you say? Oftentimes, I see people fret and change their mind. They end up opting to trim it only an inch or two, but the bold and courageous one says, "Here" and levels her hand next to her chin. The hairdresser then asks, "Are you sure?" and the woman says with conviction, "Yes!" That's the person who is ready. That's the person who is strong in her decision and has prepared herself to be ready to make the change she really wants. The fear disappears when the first pieces of hair are cut. The attachment to her long hair got severed right then and there, and although there is a tinge of pain of what was, the woman sees her hair flow piece by piece onto the floor and says quietly to herself, "Goodbye hair. It was a great run, but here comes the new me. I am ready!" When the haircut is done, especially when your eyeglasses have been off, and you are unable to see clearly, there is this fear, excitement, and anticipation of whether you love your new look or not. As you put your eyeglasses on, you start to see yourself clearly. Whether you love it or you hate it, either way, you took a step in making the change you set out to do. You will never know whether you like the new short haircut or not until you actually do it. If you stayed with your long haircut, nothing much would have changed and what you really wanted was something different.

Whenever you encounter fear, an emotion that can wreak havoc in your mind and your body, ask yourself, "What do you really want? How badly do you want this? Are you really ready to make a change in your reality or do you want to keep things the same as they are now? Does it give you a boost of energy when you think of this? Does it light your fire? How important is this for you?" Know your truth, know what you want, and make decisions from your truth about whether to take action or not.

There is something to be gained in experiencing change. Instead of nurturing the fear of change, you can always choose to grow the opportunities it brings.

Another hindrance may also be the fear of embarrassment, being different, and what people and society might say. A community can be a great source of support but can also be a tough judge in someone's decision especially if it is not the norm of the society's belief system.

We often make decisions based on society's expectation of us. We do not take into account what we want and what our soul wants. We give others' beliefs and opinions more importance over our own. Compromising what we want creates a rift in expressing our deepest desires and needs. This is a discord between your reality and your soul. Whenever there is a disconnect, it creates an imbalance and disharmony within the self. When you suppress what you are feeling and do not communicate what bothers you, you can easily lose a part of yourself. You can also feel frustrated and angry that you are unable to express yourself. All these can be felt by your body as emotions are created by the mind, generated by the body, and managed by the spirit. Your body feels what your mind and what your spirit feel.

I had been working with someone named Carol, who had difficulty expressing her thoughts and her feelings because she was afraid of being misunderstood. She had been in a volatile and verbally abusive household where her mother was an alcoholic. Carol had also just abruptly and suddenly lost her father to a heart attack. She came to me, and I noticed moments of left-sided ticking and unconscious movements. Throughout our sessions, I noticed that whenever she became uncomfortable with her emotions, these unconscious movements start to happen. I noticed that she held on to a lot of stagnant energy in her chest, which caused her to not be able to breathe deeply. Her shoulders stay raised up toward her neck and head, giving little room for her neck to be free. There was a feeling of fullness of her chest, tight and tense shoulders, and feeling like something was stuck in her throat when there was nothing there. Carol often said she felt like she had a lump in her throat. Medically, she had no illness. We worked together for many weeks on releasing this habitual blockage by finding a modality that she was comfortable working with. We talked about her goal of getting herself comfortable with her own body. As weeks passed, Carol started to learn to express herself effectively, coming from her truth. She got back her smile and was able to laugh again. I taught her specific breathing exercises that worked for her so she could manage her energy through breathing and through movement. I taught her how to gather her energy by making her core strong. We also used sound meditation through the use of singing bowls. A significant breakthrough happened when Carol was finally comfortable enough to allow herself to use her voice as a sound healing tool along with the breathing exercises. It was then that she said that there was some relief in the lump in her throat that she had felt for so long. She had been practicing her breathing exercises and learned to relax her chest through it. As the sessions progressed, I noticed that her ticking had become very rare. Her friend mentioned this as well.

It is a sense of freedom to know that you can be just yourself. Learning how to verbalize and express your truth as much as releasing your frustrations and all the heaviness you are carrying helps you be a bit more comfortable living in your own body. It is like the real you wanting to get out but can't because you are just trying to keep it together. In reality, you are actually about to burst from the inside. Medically, everything seems to be fine, but deep inside, something is already brewing. In Carol's case, she just wanted the real her to come out, wanted to be comfortable being herself. Taking action to allow that helped her move forward, and she started to find joy and appreciation in the little things in her life.

It is also as important to know when to take action as when to wait for the right moment. A gauge I use when I choose to walk away is whether or not the situation is helpful and necessary. How important is this circumstance for you? Are you willing to spend that time, energy, and effort? Is it worth it for you? Will it make a difference if you decide to take action? Or is this something your heart would rather walk away from? You will know what you need to do the closer you are to your heart and your soul.

When taking action, mindfulness is key. Being mindful means being focused and being present. It is taking action in creating harmony within the self, the environment, and humanity. It carries a healing and peaceful energy. It is movement with the energy and intention of peace. Moving with mindfulness is not only through tai chi or qi gong but can be in performing our everyday tasks. Tai chi is a Chinese martial art that is also used to harmonize and align energies within one's body. Qi gong is the movement of energy or energy dance that help coordinate breathing, posture, and meditation, and can be used for healing. Both can help in stress reduction and aim to promote health and spiritual training.

Mindfulness can be found in our everyday activities. It can be staying in one position over a long period of time, or it can be a moving meditation. Cooking can be a form of moving meditation as well as eating, walking, breathing, bathing, or dancing. It is the intention and focus you put into the action that creates a space of healing if you choose it.

When you put your loving energy and your heart's focus and happiness in what you are doing, for instance cooking, you feel contented or pleasurable and at peace. This same energy gets transferred over to your cooking. No matter how simple or complicated your recipe might be, the people who partake in your meal will feel the nourishment, not only from the nutrients from the food, but from the energy you shared in your cooking. Similar to preparing your child's lunchbox, you prepare it with so much love and affection. This is why, as a child, we always felt mom's lunch pack or meals were always the best.

When you have a goal and you take action, energy flows. When you hold it in, it becomes stagnant and creates a blockage in the flow of your own body's energy. Thinking too much, chronic overthinking, and worry without action can cause many physical manifestations. This may include headaches, chest tightness, shortness of breath, body stiffness, feeling exhausted quickly, being always tired, and having difficulty sleeping. This can happen when we allow fear to stop us from following our heart and our soul. Instead of creating anxiety from worries, move energy by taking action so the worry and overthinking can be released. Change your circumstance by taking action and overcoming your stagnant thoughts.

You have authority over your own thoughts, your own mind, and your own body. If you feel like being out of control or do not know how to manage them, do not hesitate to ask for help. Asking for help is not for the weak but for the wise. It is wise to know when to ask and receive help, especially when needed. Wanting to grow to be the best version of you is always a wise decision. It all comes down to choice and taking action in your choice.

I've worked with people who are bipolar, on medications, under treatment, who are looking to learn more about themselves. There is fear, trauma to the psyche and the emotional body as well as having a scattered and leaking energy. There is an imbalance between the mind, the body, and the spirit. I help hold the energetic space and help them to see themselves as a whole. There is a pattern that many times we do not see on our own. We need someone to help us be a mirror to who we really are in conjunction to how our energies are being utilized and how we are living our lives. Reconnecting these rifts can activate healing.

There was a lady named Amy who had been diagnosed as bipolar and was under treatment. She was very abrupt and had a rough-around-the-edges kind of approach to everyone she met, but deep down was actually a person who strove to be good and was a beautiful soul. She often saw someone else for her sessions, and this was the first time she came to a session with me. She initially resisted my service as I revealed to her that I saw red as her dominant aura color at the time. The color red represents passion and courage, a survival instinct and a strong will, but has a tendency of being vulgar, having little patience, and angers easily.

She said, "No! I am never red. I'm always blue. You're wrong!"

I replied, "I don't know what to tell you, but that is what I see."

We continued on, and I noticed how she had difficulty focusing. She started to share a bit about her life, as I saw her being a healer. She shared how she had been abused at a young age and how no one seemed to listen and understand her. She had been a survivor, and many people have actually come to see and talk to her because they knew that she understood them. There was this tenderness and toughness about her that was all a part of who she was. These opposites about herself, the yin and the yang, what she saw as good and bad, needed to be acknowledged that they were a part of the whole and not separate. I had to give extra effort in holding the energetic space during our session because I was also holding her energy so it would not get scattered and leak, as that has been her habit. We focused on gathering and holding energy through sound meditation. Toward the end of the session, she said that I was right about seeing red after all. Five minutes after our session ended, I noticed her energy changing back to the time before she came to see me. Her energy became scattered and leaking again as she talked here and there, flitting from one person to the next. She was back to acting tough and no-nonsense again. She was able to hold on for five minutes before returning to her habit. Habits take time to change. She knew she needed help and was doing her best to get better in her own way. Knowing to ask for help needs to be acknowledged and honored. That alone shows the respect and care you have for yourself.

When asking for help, it is also extremely important to be clear to express what you really want. Being ambivalent in your own feelings about not wanting your loved ones to worry about your issues but really wishing deep down that you can be understood is a disconnect. It is the dissociation between what you really want and what you 'think' you should do that might be better for others. You do not have to be the scapegoat or the sacrificial lamb in your own discomfort. You, yourself, deserve the love and understanding you so often happily give to others. In making your loved ones part of your life, which includes not only the ups but the downs as well, you can create that space of closeness—a bond and connection that is more strong and more rooted. I know for sure that your loved ones will be more than happy to be there for you. Most importantly, your heart needs to speak more than the logical mind at this time. Let the heart speak and let it be free! Be vulnerable! Be open to how you're feeling, your thoughts and worries, your fears, and your frustrations. Do not assume that your loved ones can read your mind.

Assumptions can lead to misunderstandings. Be clear in expressing what your needs are.

I love this quote from author Tatiana Amico, "Be the woman that knows what she wants, says what she wants, asks for what she wants, and goes after what she wants." Let your loved ones know exactly what you need, whether a listening ear, just someone to be with, an embrace, a cuddle, a cup of coffee or tea, a change of scenery, just to sit with you, or reassurances that you are loved and supported. Let them know that there might be days that you might be cranky, angry, or just might seem not yourself, and in that moment, that they should please ask, "Are you in pain? What can I do?" This is the time that you may want to push your loved ones away, and that can be very hurtful for them. Again, let your raw and vulnerable you speak from your heart. "I'm in a lot of pain right now, and I just don't know what to do with myself. I just want to lay down and rest by myself," or, "Can you just give me a loving hug, please?" or, "I'm so tired right now; I just need you to hold me please." Express your needs and what you are feeling. Being vulnerable does not mean you are helpless or weak. Being vulnerable can mean knowing when you need help and when you are brave enough to show the raw part of you. Vulnerability does not have to mean weakness. It can also be wisdom and courage from within from sharing that part of you.

Know that you have the power over your own body, your own life. You get to choose how you want to live it. You can create your own circumstance through your choices and actions. If you do not desire where you are right now, then move to change your situation. Choose to take action in creating your own reality. No one else can live your life for you. Only you can make your life the way you want, however you want.

When you take action, not only is being mindful important but so is doing your absolute best. Give it your all—your 100%. Whether it works out or you find that it is not for you, you will live without looking back with, "What if I did this?" or "If only I did that." You only live this life once, so do give it your all. You cannot go back to yesterday but you can live fully in your today. This is your moment. You have the now and this time and space to be your very best. When you create a habit of doing your best and being the authentic version of you, it will eventually become effortless. You will learn to not overthink and doubt your yesterdays.

In some of my relationships, whether it be boyfriend, an ex, or passing friends, I give it my all especially when there is a misunderstanding or a disconnect. I believe that come what may, whatever the outcome may be, wherever it may lead is where it needs to be. I do not look back and tell myself what else could I have done because I knew I gave it my best.

Moving forward, living a life of being your 100%, doing your ultimate best, in the moment that is now, is one of the most freeing experience. You can let go of the what-ifs, if-onlys, and the maybes if you gave it your all. You may not feel it right at that exact moment, but you will be able to see later on how your decision to give it your 100% will give you a sense of freedom and leave no room for regrets.

"Do your best and live with no regrets!"

Forgiveness and being thankful are also your superpowers. They say love can move mountains. I say forgiveness and thankfulness are the children of love. They are the superkids of love. Grow your capacity to forgive just like how children forgive. Do you ever notice that children forgive more easily and tend to not hold grudges? They just want to play well together with their new friends, be joyful, and enjoy each other's company. They generally tend to help and encourage each other. We need to learn from them, living and enjoying in the moment with big hearts and a forgiving soul.

We often easily forgive others but are extremely hard on ourselves. Do not be too hard on yourself. Forgive yourself as you are not perfect.

Not being perfect gives us room to grow. Letting go of anger, regret, guilt, shame, blame, and negativity directed inward to ourselves releases the shackles of self-harm and promotes the beauty of self-healing and acceptance. Knowing that our emotions are related to our physical body, why punish and harm yourself? What good will that do to you? Instead, you can always choose to be thankful to have the opportunity to grow and better yourself. Mistakes can happen. They are the opportunities for growth. If the mistake is unintentionally repeated, it only means we need to keep practicing until we learn to move away from our habits or patterns in dealing with things. It is simply a part of growing.

Gratefulness is a trait that can help you strengthen your character. Whenever you have difficulties in life, look on these as big opportunities to grow yourself. The larger the challenge, the bigger the growth. You will have little or no growth if it comes too easily. Additionally, learning something new can help prevent dementia and can activate new neural connections in your brain. This is called neuroplasticity. Gone is the days old saying, "You cannot teach old dogs new tricks." Apparently, that is untrue.

Again, our body has its own healing capability for our optimal well-being. You can choose not to limit yourself to what seems to be the norm, but know instead that you can choose to be the person you want to be and move to live the life you want to live. It's about stepping up, stepping forward, and taking action toward where you want to be and who you want to be in your own life.

Create a habit of healing, a habit of growth, and a habit of listening to your heart and your soul. The more you practice this, the more you will see that you are getting closer to the life you are meant to live, the life you are looking for. Your body will naturally feel this shift, and you may feel effortless transformation happen within your whole being. This was the case with me throughout this process.

Take ownership of your life and be responsible for your actions. I cannot emphasize enough that a shift and transformation in your life to a life of growth, healing, and freedom of the mind, body, and soul is not just for the numbered few but for everyone and anyone who chooses it sincerely and who moves toward it through mindful actions.

Chapter 8
STEP 4—Act to Inspire & Motivate

As you take your life into your own hands and your healing into your own life, you are going to need support. The best support you always have when you cannot feel the hand guiding you from above, from God, the universe or divinity, is actually right in front of you. It's you! You have within you the divinity, God, the universe. That is why we pray to connect.

You need to learn to be your own cheerleader. Be your own best friend and most especially the best fan and lover you will ever have. Treat yourself well and uplift your spirits. Why wait for others to boost your spirit when you are right there to help? Why is it okay to help others and not okay to help yourself? You absolutely can, and it is most definitely okay!

When you hit a road block, be the one who says, "You can do this! Let's figure this out. This is in front of us for a reason. Let's work through it. You got this!"

Do not listen to the little old limiting you who will try to give up and tell you that you are not good enough. There will be a part of you that will try to backtrack and go back to what it is comfortable even when the past had created unhappiness and disharmony within yourself. Refuse to sabotage your own self and your own happiness.

Challenge yourself, but do not be too hard on yourself. Mistakes are absolutely okay. They are the best way to learn. Be confident in making mistakes and be confident in finding ways to rectify them. If one way does not work, try another. This helps exercise your brain.

Give no room for the blame and shame duo. This will just stunt your progress unnecessarily. These can hurt your psyche as much as they can hurt your physical body. If you did your best and it did not work out, move on by finding another way. Wallowing in blame or shame will not get you anywhere. If it causes you harm, let it go. If it heals, then let it in.

Live simply. Know your priorities and focus your energy there. Learning to manage your energy is also learning to manage your body's health. Know that what you put out will come right back around. It is the karmic cycle, the universal truth. When something needs to be changed, then change it. When something needs to be moved, then move it. When something needs to be thrown away, then throw it away. When something needs to be added, then add it. Take action accordingly with love and mindfulness. Follow your heart!

There is no time for excuses. If you want it, just go get it. No matter the how, find a way. If you really want it, you will move mountains. You have the power and the capability. Take down the blockages you have put up in stopping yourself to fully reach your dreams.

In my experience, there was a time that I faced my own blockage and my own belief and preconception. I really asked myself what I wanted. I asked whether or not I was ready for this, and my answer was, "Yes, I need to be ready because this is my reason for living. I finally know my life's purpose, and there is no reason to waste time anymore."

I remember when I started this journey of helping others with their healing and growing into themselves. I had been very conservative as to who I wanted to help. I only looked to help those who were associates, friends, or family of those I already knew. The time came when I felt stuck and felt like things needed to move. Things didn't seem to feel quite right and where I wanted it to be. I realized that I wasn't really exercising my full potential. My goal is to be of service to as many people who desperately want to know more about themselves and help connect what is happening to them on the outside with what is being reflected by their inside. I decided to have a real sit down and chat with myself. It was then that I found out that I haven't been stepping up. I had been hiding behind the fear of being known. "Why?," I asked myself. Being well known and popular carries a lot of responsibility. I had other responsibilities but this responsibility of fully making my life's purpose into my life's work was a serious matter to me. I knew that there would be many extraordinary shifts that would happen in my life when I fully chose to take this on as my life's work, the reason I was living and breathing. I've learned that one of my greatest happiness is to see people being empowered in restoring true joy in their life and fully embracing who they are. Facing myself made me realize that I had blocked my own dreams with fear. My fear overshadowed my desire to reach my goals. I realized that I needed to embrace and be okay with being known and popular because that was the way to impact many people's lives, to hear the message of healing and happiness. I know that this message should not only be for a numbered few. We are all in this together, and what better way than to help each other grow into healing, hope, and happiness?

It is a great joy of mine to be of service and help others transform their lives to be the people they want to be and live the lives they want to live. This is my reason for living, so here I am stepping up and stepping forward, ready, and taking action toward my dream.

Have a real honest talk with yourself. Give yourself advice as you would give your best friend. Your friends tell you that you are the best at helping them. Why not be the best friend to yourself?

Give yourself hugs and kisses galore as you would your lover. In moments of feeling low and depressed, know that you are never alone. You are supported. You will come out of it and grow stronger. You will not always feel this way. It will pass and you will be alright.

You may feel frustrated if you do not reach your goal or it becomes extremely hard to get there. You can have many kinds of emotions come up. Learn to watch your emotions and see where they start, how they travel throughout your body and how you and your body react to them. Utilize your emotions as your personal power tools to grow yourself.

Be honest with yourself. Do not say "Yes" when you really mean "No." Communicate your truth by speaking from your heart, free of malice or harmful emotions. Be gracious and kind. It is okay to ask for help. You do not need to do everything yourself. It is easier to grow when you are around like-minded people who share your struggles and accept you for who you are.

Check in with yourself and make sure you are treated well by you. Do not allow energies that aim to harm come to affect you. Only receive what is good. Checking in gives you space to connect and acknowledge where you are in your life right now, whether or not you are in alignment with your truth and whether you are living the life you have designed for yourself.

There is no need to impress anyone or prove yourself to anybody. You are the one who gets to exclusively live your life. Therefore, only you have the right and get a legitimate say about it. Others have their own lives to take care of. You have yours. Let others worry about theirs, and you take care of yours. Many people focus too much outside themselves and have a lot of time criticizing others because oftentimes they are too afraid to look within themselves and scared of what they might find.

Allow others who want to support your growth be a part of your life. Just keep in mind that you are still the leader of this fan base. You are the ultimate and forever loyal fan who never gives up on their rock star, the rock star that is you.

Be your own role model. Be your own rock star. Give yourself the platform to be free to express your vulnerability and authenticity. Learn ways to empower yourself. Whenever you feel you are about to give up, remind yourself of the commitment you made. Remember the moment when you had the clarity in your decision. Know that this can be just a bump on the road you need to pass through and that it will get better.

Know that where you are right now and what you are going through is happening or has happened to others as well. Send them encouragement as you would send yourself.

Learn words or phrases that brighten your day or uplift your spirit. Create your own words of encouragement or your own cheer. Here are some examples you can use:

- "You can do this!"
- "You got this!"
- "No worries. Everything will work out the way it is meant to."
- "You're okay. You're alright."
- "It's okay. Let's take a breath and try again."
- "You're doing great. Keep going."

- "I am the epitome of love and will pour all the love in everything that I do."
- "I am the master of my life and have the power to choose how I want to live it."
- "I choose to be the light and choose to greet the light in every person I meet."
- "Don't worry; be happy." –Bob Marley

Take good care of your body and spend more time with yourself, free from distractions such as your cellphone or the internet.

Do not feel bad if you cannot do something for someone or meet with anyone when you have a date with yourself. You are important too. Placing yourself first is okay, and there is nothing to be sorry or feel guilty about that.

Learn to not only love your body but to be in love with your body and your whole being. Be the most beautiful thing you ever saw on this planet. Treat yourself as the most beautiful creature you ever laid eyes on. Honor and respect this grand beauty. When you believe in your own beauty and worth, the way you treat yourself will be different. The way you will treat others will change as well. When you are able to see your beauty, including your scars and pock marks, you are able to see others' beauty and who they really are behind those scars, pock marks, sarcasms, and hurtful words. You will find that they are not separate from you at all. They are similar and closer to who you really are. We are mirrors of our own self. Who you see in front of you can be a reflection of who you are. Often, we hate something about somebody only to realize that we are somewhat like that too. What we hate in others is oftentimes what we hate about ourselves.

Know that sometimes healing requires wading in your own pool of yuck and muck. It is necessary to get to know your aches, your pains, your frustrations, and all the feelings that get you down. You may need a nice long chat with your Ego, and be in your discomfort. Get comfortable in your own discomfort to figure out together what needs to be done. Grab a drink with your preconceptions and judgements of yourself. This process may not be pretty, but it is necessary. When you feel these things, it can be overwhelming. You may sometimes want to give up and go back to what was easy and the life that you have been used to. You may want to go back to your comfort zone. Remind yourself of your promise and that going back will just bring you back to the same thing and the same place before choosing to take action in this journey of growth and healing. Encourage your own self. Be firm and grow in your conviction. Be your own inspiration and your own motivation to be the person you want to be and live the life you want to live. This shows the respect, care, love, and attention that you are giving to yourself and your body's needs.

Create a balance in your way of life. This means being able to do the things you love and staying true to yourself while integrating life outside of the 'you' and not be overwhelmed. Let's say you have a scale. On one end are the three aspects of your body: mind, body, and spirit. The other consists of work, school, family, relationships, responsibilities, time for church, gym, meetings, housing, car, food, etc.

Find what is important to put on your scale and what to let go. Find what makes you whole and what makes your spirit strong. Know what you need to balance. Figure out what balance is for you. Balance is important in managing your life.

A bright and pure energy is important in balance. It is what you need to keep going. Nurture and grow a pure and bright energy. Take time to replenish and recharge yourself to be ready to take on anything that comes into your life. Being aware of yourself and what your body needs is crucial in the process of growth and healing.

Live to keep your spirit alive. Keep the fires of passion burning, the light of life. If you feel it dimming, find your balance, and rekindle and grow that passion and will for life. You are where you need to be at this very moment. Sometimes, you need to stop by a pit stop along the way in your journey to self and healing. This temporary stopover may be necessary to gather and replenish energy or learn something that you need to continue for your journey. Find your passion and live your spirit's passion. This can inspire and motivate you to be your own source of energy—your own zest for life.

Pain can be your friend and your guide. Be not afraid of pain. It is telling you something important. Pain in your body can be a call to listen inward. Be not afraid of getting hurt; it is when you can also learn what true encompassing love means. Do not be afraid to be yourself; it is what you and others strive for.

Messages come in many forms. It can be from a dream or from an accident. It can be in nature, or it can be in our own body. Be vigilant to all the messages in and all around you. As you actively watch for these, you will notice many things that you have taken for granted. As you open yourself up to all that is good, you will find that the puzzle pieces of your life will come in its place and things will make sense.

It was after the two car accidents that I had in 2016 that I had to really have a serious and good look at my life. By the second accident, I asked, "Is this a message for me? What are you trying to tell me?" I thought I was happy with my work as a nurse and working with children at the yoga center. I had been busy throughout the week focused on these things, along with spending quality time with my boyfriend and family. I had reveled in being busy, and I was happy doing so. Due to the accidents, I had been out of work for almost a year, and I started to feel frustration and could see depression slowly creeping in. It really forced me to reflect on my life and where I was heading, what future I had designed for myself living versus the life I was living at that time. This was the time I became serious with my soul searching, becoming more detailed and specific about what I wanted from my life. I went on a spiritual journey and on a vision quest. I realized that the accumulation of life lessons and all the trainings I have been through since I was born, but most especially since 2006, were a step closer to where I am now. In my reflection, I remembered that four years prior, I had asked for guidance from God and the universe that if by this time my life was not where it needed to be, to show me the way, even if it was necessary to be jarred from my life. This memory had been completely buried in the back of my mind. Once things became clear to me and I started to take action to live my life's dream, things moved quickly. Many things happened in less than a year's time. My body was not how it used to be before the accidents, my aunt who was like a mother to me abruptly and unexpectedly passed away, my eight-plus-year relationship with my boyfriend started to show its cracks and abruptly ended, and I finally reunited with my estranged father who I had cut ties with for about twenty years. All this time, I was back at work as a nurse full time, and I was also studying acupuncture full time, funding school on my own. In addition, as an alternative healer, I was also working with those who needed help with healing. Through all these, my intuition became stronger as I gained and grew many gifts.

Make changes in the things you want to improve within yourself. Be persistent until you accomplish your goal. When you want something badly enough, you will move mountains to get it. If you cannot move the mountain yourself, whatever it takes, you will find a way to get it to move like your life depends on it. This is why there is a saying, "If there's a will, there's a way." Be resilient in achieving your goal.

There is no time for feeling sorry for yourself. No time for self-pity. Get busy in moving toward the direction of light and love. Do not allow yourself to limit your own gifts and abilities. Know that you are born with all that you need to fulfill your life's dream.

There is something empowering about making your choice and taking action. It gives you a sense of ownership and accountability for your life. You can move your life however you want. This reality is the freedom you seek. You just need to go for it. Encourage yourself to never give up and to do your best. You will reach your goal with dedication and conviction. Move with love and live with love.

Choose to grow your character. Live with honesty and integrity. Obstacles come your way to strengthen your character. It is an opportunity to be thankful for all the challenges, teachers, and lessons that come your way. Everything that comes to you, whether difficult for you or not, has a deeper meaning and has a deeper purpose for you. Trust that the things beyond your control or out of your hands are meant to be what they are. Know that if you do not understand them now, one day every piece of your life will come together and fit. You will understand when it is time.

Someone close to me initially underwent the process of finding out her unknown illness and did not understand why her abdomen started swelling, which caused her to have difficulty breathing. This was sixty-eight-year-old Mandy, who later on found out that the cause of her abdominal swelling was due to a rare type of cancer. I saw the color gray as her aura, like her life force was slowly disappearing. On a metaphysical and energetic level, I sensed that it was all a culmination of her life and everything she held in. I recall having one number that came up in my mind and asked Mandy, "What happened to you at eighteen years old that was significant to you? Something happened that changed the course of your life." I could see the wall she had put up even as we were having the session. She finally gave in and spoke about her boyfriend who she genuinely loved and cared for at the time. She had felt betrayed by this boyfriend, and this was when I saw the spark in her spirit started to dim as she decided to stay with her own family. Mandy was very much loved and cared for throughout her life. She never married and had no children of her own. There were many things she wanted to do but chose not to, focusing on others especially her family and her loved ones. Many people confided in her as she knew how to find solutions for their concerns. She gave good advice, was empathetic, and could truly connect with people easily. Mandy had the ability to make you feel better and make you feel that everything will be alright. She was trustworthy, loyal, hardworking, and found simple pleasures in life such as eating and spending time with friends and family. I was relieved to know that Mandy did process and digest what we covered in the session. Her sister Laura came to me and shared that Mandy confided in her everything she was holding within herself. Mandy revealed the many things that concerned her, affected her, and worried her. She shared even what she thought of as forgotten past that still had a great effect on her emotions. She never spoke to anyone about how she felt or what she kept for so long until then. Mandy had been carrying all these by herself for many years. This was about fifty years of her life that were finally released and brought to light. Mandy's condition, however, quickly turned for the worst, and she eventually and abruptly passed away. Her life force could not sustain her body's condition anymore. On her final day, she was at peace and was ready to move on. Mandy actually came to me in a dream soon after she passed away and gave me advice and encouragement to reach more people like her when she was alive. She has been an inspiration and a motivation for me to continue and expand the work that I do.

Chapter 9
STEP 5—Receiving (Achieve, Accomplish & The Art of Receiving)

W hen you are on the journey to healing, when you have a goal and a destination, you sometimes get sidetracked. Be vigilant of distractions that might confuse you and could make you forget that you have a destination to get to. Be mindful and check on yourself every day. See where you are. When left unchecked, we can easily get lost and lose a part of ourselves.

Watch your feelings and how your body reacts. Follow through with achieving your dream of health, happiness, and peace. Even with struggle and effort, when you know what you want, you will go for it, and nothing should stop you, not even your own self.

You are actually the most challenging person you need to befriend and love. You are the one who will either oppose your own self or support yourself. Do not give yourself too much of a hard time; forgive,

87

and work on moving forward. Watch your habits on how you treat yourself. Practice in aligning and connecting all aspects of your body— your mind, body, and spirit.

When I was brought up, I was taught to always be kind and good to others. Taking care of others first became what was acceptable. Although that is a good thing, it becomes unhealthy when it creates an imbalance with taking care of your own self. I ended up creating a habit of focusing on my work, my responsibilities, and my patients without being aware of what I myself needed. I only remember after the fact. It is often when your body starts feeling something out of the ordinary that you start to realize that you need to take care of it.

When I was working in the Medical Surgical Unit, I often skipped meals or delayed them indefinitely. I did not get a chance to drink much water, especially since we were not allowed to have it with us while working. Nurses on the Medical Surgical unit are on their feet the majority of their entire work shift. Although I had heard that nurses are often predisposed or later on develop some type of digestive issues such as ulcers or UTIs (Urinary Tract Infection), I still did what I did because of the sense of responsibility for my patients.

As a younger nurse, I had the stamina and the physical ability to sustain this, but as I got older, I started to feel different. I ended up working the day shift because I never really had any sleep pattern working in the night time. It all depended on my work schedule and my days off. I never really thought at first about how it impacted my physical life.

The first few times I returned to work, I would feel like a truck just hit my entire body. I felt like I had just gone throughout the day at work and barely survived a tsunami. I never realized how much wear and tear working as a nurse takes on the physical body. I realized that I had been doing this and exposed to this way of life for so many years that my body perceived it as a norm. To cope in environments such as this, multitasking and being in charge of the many aspects of care for their patients, nurses hold the space of healing for the patients and their families. They also hold the space in keeping the environment in harmony along with collaborating with all other personnel they work with. They juggle many things and act to balance it all. With all these, all aspects of the body are under stress in holding this space and fulfilling these responsibilities. Nurses are often excellent caretakers of others but not so good when it comes to taking care of themselves.

It is wise that as soon as you get home, you get to unwind. But in most cases, people come home and have more responsibilities to take care of, especially when there are children involved. It is even more so when you are an only parent. Take time off and time to slow down. You deserve some rest and relaxation in between your lifestyle of constant and never-ending obligations. You definitely deserve some self-care.

In times of the habit of a fast-paced life, it is important to take a break to recharge, recalibrate, replenish, and rejuvenate. You are deserving of a quality of life. Get quality rest, quality sleep, eat quality food, quality everything. Know that you deserve the absolute best.

Exercise living with quality. Schedule in a time in your day to check in with yourself—be it a minute or more, an hour or so. Choose to take time to care for yourself. Let go of what tenses your muscles, organs, and body—the stressors in your life. You can always get back to those stressors after your time with resting and relaxing.

Release what occupies your mind during your rest. Choose to have nothing get in the way of your relaxation time, especially from your own self—your own thoughts and emotions. It is important to take time to feel good about yourself by just being in the present.

Go on vacations or just take a break from your own life, away from all worries and overthinking. Avoid bringing or holding on to anything that busies or burdens your mind, body, and spirit. Try not to bring with you or think about paperwork and bills. Try to take care of these before or after your time off. Do not bring in other things during your "You" time. Distracting yourself by focusing on other things instead of focusing inward toward yourself causes you to lose some of your energy. Focusing inward is actually a way to receive and replenish abundant energy.

Do not feel guilty and embrace the 'me-first' and the 'me-too' mentality so long as you fully understand the responsibility behind it. When you are in alignment with your whole being, you will find that things will just automatically fall into place. Do you notice that the times when you are happy, your day seems to just be going on the trajectory of bountiful blessings? It is easier to see and meet the beauty of everyone and everything around you.

I worked with a man named Jarod who was fifty-eight years old. He had been married and had two kids who are now adults. He and his wife, Jane, had been separated for five years and lived in separate dwellings but tried to remain friends despite the underlying discomfort for the sake of their children. Jane had initially been the breadwinner who started a lucrative business of import/export. Jarod eventually became an integral part of Jane's business, and all was well for a time. Due to many misunderstandings, they eventually separated, and Jarod decided to start his own import/export business similar to Jane's. He was often told that he would never be successful because Jane was really the brain and the driving force of the success of the company. Jarod strove to prove them wrong and is now successful on his own. He is now able to have some free time to spend with himself and his friends because he was able to hire more people to work in his business. As he had more time, he started to get treatments to maintain his youthful look. He started to travel all over the world and purchased luxury things for himself. However, this eventually was not what fully satisfied or solved his underlying unease.

Jarod came to see me not knowing what to expect, but he just knew that something did not feel right. He always felt exhausted despite having more time for himself. I had been referred to him by someone we both knew, but he only chose to reach out to me months later.

Jarod was prepared and open to anything that could shed light on his dilemma of not knowing what was wrong. As I guided him through clearing and cleansing, I saw how deep his loneliness was. Jarod often spent time with his friends but never really felt fully understood. He felt like he could not fully reveal all of himself to them. He was afraid of being misunderstood and had a fear of being seen as a misfit in the group. He did not want to burden them with his 'I don't know what the problem is, but there is something not right in my life' issue. He wanted to be the great friend, the positive person, and the pillar of support to his friends. Jarod felt most safe and more at ease being alone in the sanctuary he had made as his home. This was where he felt comfortable being his truest self. Without judgement or criticism, he could just be himself.

Jarod was a very giving person by nature. He enjoyed sharing his abundance without expecting anything in return. This was often misunderstood by others as showing off, and this was actually very hurtful for Jarod. However, he could not just sit back and do nothing when he knew he had the capacity to help someone, so he endured the criticisms.

Jarod chose to continue to work hard and live in comfort of luxury, but his happiness seemed to be disappearing slowly. Going deeper, I helped him realize that he had not acknowledged and valued his own worth. He was still striving for success when he had already reached his goal. He was already successful with a thriving business. He realized that he was still living his life trying to prove that Jane was not the only one who could run a business and make it into a success. So I asked, "Why are you working so hard to prove that you are already where you are?" It already is a given, and there is proof of that. "Why is Jane's opinion of you so important over your own?" He had put Jane on an unreachable pedestal that he was trying to reach despite the clear fact that he had already reached there long ago.

I encouraged Jarod to shower himself with all the love and affection he would a lover. He deserved happiness and all good things in life. I suggested that he have a date with himself and truly do the things that he enjoyed, not caring what others may think, make himself feel how special and how precious he was in his own life. He chose his path and made his own road a success just as he had set out to do. That deserved to be honored and acknowledged. He deserved to be celebrated for who he was and all he had done. I helped him realize that he needed to give back to himself and love himself again.

Exercising self-love and really embracing and feeling self-worth as your own are essential in growing in strength and confidence to be true to who you are with no apologies.

When you are in pain and feel exhausted, know that many times you may realize that what you need most is to feel love, support, and affection. Allow this to be a part of your life instead of using your defenses and rational thoughts to push people away. Sometimes, it is simply what we need, and we are deserving of that. We are deserving of love, support, care, and affection. We are deserving of all that is good.

Taking excellent care of yourself and loving yourself is extremely important. This is absolutely necessary in order to optimally take excellent care of others as well. The mindset of "others before self" needs to be readjusted. Once you learn what true respect toward your own self is, you will see that your perception of taking care of others is not separate but one and the same as taking care of yourself. There is no difference. The more you focus on the outside and not taking care of the inside, the more you create a disconnect from your true self.

Reward yourself and take time to celebrate. Celebrate your accomplishments and your milestones. More importantly, celebrate the awesomeness that is you! You deserve to be celebrated, especially by you. You have made it this far, have accomplish and achieved many things, and persevered through tough times. You have been amazing and definitely deserve a celebration. This is not only reserved for your birthday, but you can choose to celebrate any time of the year. I often look forward to celebrations because they are an uplifting time. We need happiness in our lives, and what better way than creating that for yourself? It is the happiness and peace that come from the inside that are lasting.

When you know and experience this truth, you will find that you do not have to look very far for the answers you are looking for. Sometimes, you may just need help in shining a light into your own self to find it. It is like going to your attic or basement looking for something. You need light to see clearly.

Do not worry about what others think. With the worry of money and the opinion of others aside, reflect on what you really want and be sure that you are heading in the direction of where you want to go. These two often determine the decisions we make and the direction we are headed. We often like to go with the flow and go where everyone is going. We do this because we want to belong, to be accepted and be one with society. We follow what everyone else is doing because it does not require as much effort as compared to flowing in our own direction, the direction of our soul.

Get into the habit of chatting with yourself and really take into sincere consideration what the inside you is saying. When you shut that part of you, you become unhappy and feel lacking or like something is missing. This was the cause of my midlife-like crisis at seventeen/eighteen years old. That something missing is the disconnect with the inner you because of being busy going along with everyone else and just accomplishing what you feel is expected of you. A balance between your inner world and your outer world needs to happen. What you feel inside can be reflected by how your body feels. Consequently, what you feel inside reflects what you do on the outside.

It is vital that you also know how to receive as much as you also give. When you notice that you become uncomfortable receiving thanks or appreciation for all the you do, for touching people's hearts, for being thoughtful, and for just being you, it means you have not fully embraced others' love and appreciation. There needs to be an exchange so you do not feel exhausted. When someone constantly takes and takes from you, you will eventually get tired, and it could affect your physical body. You also deserve all the love and the care and the effort you put out and share to others. Embrace that. It is also food for your soul. Learn to not be hard on yourself, and embrace the love of others as your own.

When someone offers their appreciation and their heart to you, step up and receive it wholeheartedly. Say "You're welcome." Do not avoid it or devalue it by saying, "It is nothing." There is no need to sidestep a hug or thanks. Walk into it humbly and confidently. How would you feel if you wanted to share your heart and love to someone, and they just tapped it away on the side, saying, "It's alright, I don't need it"? It is their way of showing appreciation and thoughtfulness. They are trying to connect their hearts with you, so you should really consider connecting yours with them.

Relearning what homeostasis is, what the normal flow of your body is, is extremely important to go back in a state of zero, the original state of being. This is a state where healing can be felt. When your body is stressed and tensed up, it creates contraction and constriction. When this happens, it can form energetic blockages or stagnation. These can manifest into something solid. Manifestations from nothing to something is how I would describe this. It may cause insomnia, fatigue, pain, a feeling of 'something does not feel right' but not knowing what, inflammation or skin issues of unknown origin, feeling uncomfortable in your own body, and many more manifestations.

The way I look at it is that if you are able to move away from homeostasis, then that means you can move back into it. If you can manifest nothing into something, then you can also manifest something back into nothing. Sometimes, however, it can become a permanent fixture, and damage may have already occurred when it has been there for a very long time, as can be seen with the physical body. This does not mean you cannot achieve your optimum well-being. Know that you can still choose to be the best that you can be even at this state.

Effort is needed to make a new habit—the habit of returning to homeostasis. When your body recognizes what normal is and when you become aware and conscious of your own body and how you live, you will more quickly know when something is amiss. The faster you catch it, the earlier you can remedy it.

You see, for most of us, we did not really grow up learning about these things. We were never really taught or guided to look for answers within. It became a norm to always seem to look outward for answers or solutions. Due to my circumstances and the unrest of my soul's search, I went through many trainings, trials, and errors until I learned through experience and feeling. I realized that what I had been through and all the knowledge, wisdom, intuition, and gifts I had nourished were all not new. It had already been there for countless generations. We were just not taught or made aware of it. Our society does not often touch on this subject—inner awareness. The more you become aware of both your inner and outer self, you become aware of others with a deeper understanding. You will learn the priorities in your life and see that what is happening in your outside world can be a reflection of what is going through on your inside.

You have your own intuition just like I have mine. I chose to nurture and grow my intuition, which is the how and the why I do what I do. I learned to embrace the intangible and the unexplainable that intuition comes with. You have it too. You and I are not much different. This is also why we are mirrors to each other's souls. As you grow to know more about yourself, you will realize that you are infinite in possibilities and gifts. You will find that you are the person you need the most to create a change not only in your life but the lives of others and the whole world.

My greatest dream is for you to see yourself clearly, experience your own self, receive and hear your own messages, activate and grow your intuition and gifts, come into your own wisdom and higher self, and ultimately come into your own being. Empower yourself to be the person you want to be and live the life you dream of. Be who you are meant to be. This path may not be an easy path to take, but it can be fulfilling and freeing. Anyone can do it. All these are possible when you sincerely choose it and simply just do it.

Chapter 10
Obstacles—Past Attachments

Our past up to our present has been an adventurous ride. We have grown to who we are right now because of what we have been through, where we have been, and the people we have met.

When you grew up poor, barely meeting your basic needs, or when you grew up without a father or a mother, it can be very hard to stand on your own. You learned to depend on yourself more than you depend on others. You learned to be frugal and spend only on necessities. You became hardworking and had the conviction to emerge victorious from your status to a life of comfort and security as well as the acknowledgement of your existence. You had to sacrifice your needs and desires over your family members who needed the food to eat, place to sleep, and pieces of clothing to wear.

Being away from your loved ones or not having much time with your children due to work was necessary to reach a goal of a better future for you and your family. Risks and opportunities had to be taken to reach your dream of creating a life of comfort and abundance for your family, especially your kids. Your children become your life and your reason for living. You will do anything and everything to ensure their safety and happiness. Your life revolves around them.

As you reach your goal of living comfortably and being able to provide for your family, you may have started saving things such as memorabilia from your past and even things in the present mainly because you had been lacking in the past. The thought is that just in case you become without again, you have a backup so you will not be lacking. You do not want to be back in the situation you were in in the past. However, this can be seen as hoarding as well. There needs to be a balance between what you need at present and what to set aside for emergencies. When there is too much clutter around you, most times, that's how much clutter that can occupy in your brain. Inversely, what you feel on the inside will reflect on what is on the outside. This is an example of the internal/external connection or manifestations. The same with the physical body. What you feel on the inside can easily reflect and spill over to the external, which is the manifestation in your physical body.

You may have gone through pain and suffering from being abused and bullied at a very young age and that may even continue to adulthood, humiliated for being different from everyone else, making you feel stupid, feeling abandoned and neglected, having to be far away from your children and miss out on seeing them grow up, and even having to deal with the headache and heartache of betrayal from a cheating husband or partner. All these prompted you to build a wall that serves as a fortress around you.

As you keep getting hurt, you continue to build more walls, stronger and bigger than the last. Your soul wants to be set free, but you are afraid to bare it openly and let it go out into the world because you are afraid of getting hurt again. You have been betrayed and hurt so many times over that it is difficult for you to give your full trust to anyone. All you know is that it is only you whom you can fully depend on.

Growing up, if your parents have been absent in the majority of your upbringing due to either having to work far away or work long hours, or even losing your parents at a young age, you do your best to emulate what you believe love is. You piece together the kindness, compassion, and love you experienced from those who you saw as a mother or father figure while your own parents are away. You try your best in your own understanding and share that with your own children.

Keep watch because later on you may turn out to be very sensitive to what people say and get hurt easily, or you can be apathetic and live blandly with little emotional connection. The extremes on either side create an imbalance. You need to find the balance and prevent losing the real you.

You may also have to deal with a controlling nature from those who brought you up. People who are controlling often use manipulation to get their way. Most times, it is because they are afraid that you might get hurt, and when you get hurt, they will get hurt. It could also be just because they want their way for their own selfish reasons, their Ego liking the feel of power over another person. They may say things to make you feel bad so you will do what they want.

Being in this environment may have inspired you to prepare and be resilient so that one day, you will walk away from this situation and will never do the same to your own family and your own future. You were able to push through and emerge with a stronger willpower. This was the will to be able to forge your own path in life. You worked hard to move away from this environment of control. You took chances and made efforts to exit this reality and were able to choose and create another.

You are a survivor and a fighter, resilient in your conviction of life. This is what kept your hope alive along with the numbered few who showed you love and acknowledged your humanity. You almost gave up many times but never did because of your strong faith in God.

The many negative words, thoughts, and actions aimed at you during your upbringing were fuel to your rebellious nature. You knew this was not true and not you. So this stoked your fire in proving them wrong. However, at the same time, there could be a high likelihood that you may start believing what they were saying as true at some point. The more something is being repeated, the more likely it can be believed. It is almost akin to brainwashing. You may start believing this especially when you get exhausted of your situation, when nothing seems to go your way and you feel like giving up.

Many times, in situations like this, people say hurtful words because they make them feel better when they feel superior. It could also be because they want to convince you to do what they want. There is a possibility that they are under a lot of stress, not really knowing what they are doing, and just being strict to appear like they have everything under control. It is to hide their insecurities. It could also be that in their own way, they believe that they are doing their best. It could also most likely be that this is what they experienced in the past and believe to be a form of love, so this is what they demonstrate. There are many ways of looking at things.

Whatever the reason is, it is not in your hands. Your life is what is in your hands. What you believe about yourself, what information you want to accept as true, and what to discard are all in your power. These are all in your hands. You actually have the choice of what to download and what not to as well as what to delete in your hard drive—the hard drive being you and your life.

Your past can definitely catch up with you if you have not processed it well. If you are not aware of the lessons you needed to learn, teachers and situations will repeat themselves until you see and understand the lessons to be learned.

Growing up, I had been told that I was stupid. I had also been abused physically, mentally, and emotionally. This was not always the case, but when it was, I created a wall around me. At some point, I learned to numb out pain. I became apathetic and had difficulty forming a closeness with people the way I know I am capable of. I often hid many things from others and kept many things to myself, especially when I had doubts that I would not be understood. Even when I appeared friendly, I knew deep down that there was a wall and a disconnect.

When in my twenties, I remember a time when I was very angry at my sister for not following me, and I kicked a locked door so hard it almost came off. I had been doing kung-fu classes at the time. Thankfully, I came to my senses and thought, "You can calm down, or you can keep this up. You almost kicked the door off and almost broke it. If you break this door, you have to buy another one, spend a day waiting to get someone to come fix it, and clean up the mess." Even as I was fuming with anger, I realized how much work I would have to put in for just one moment of expressing anger in a destructive way. Not only would it inconvenience me and cost me money, but I was also being very manipulative. I do not remember what I was angry about at the time, but I do know that it was not that important. It was not a life or death situation. No one was dying, and the house was not on fire. I was the only one starting the fire.

As I calmed down, I realized that I had started showing a trait that I vowed I would never do in my future. I had transcribed a little of my own upbringing into that moment. I never wanted to grow up to be the person I did not want to be and yet, here I was doing exactly that. From that time on, I searched for a better way to express anger. I held anger in and went through a phase of being passive aggressive. I found that it does not work well for me. It caused a lump on my throat and a tightness in my body. What worked and was the best way for me was to speak my truth, share what I feel with honesty and without Ego. Finding the real reason why you are angry is the key. That is how you know if it was your Ego or the real you. Speak from your heart. When you do, it gets processed and released from your body.

Unknown to you, you are actually admired by many due to all your accomplishments and how you have lived and overcome all that you had to go through. You have proven to yourself and others the leaps and bounds, the risks and trials you had to make to be in a position to provide all that you and your family needs and so much more.

You tend to prioritize others' needs ahead of your own, especially your children's. You take better care of them and others than you take care of yourself. You are willing to sacrifice all of you for the sake of others. It becomes second nature to disregard your own self when others are involved, especially when it is your own children. Not being able to take proper care of yourself can take a toll on your physical and energy body. At some point, it can catch up to you if you are not mindful. You may start to feel aches and pains, feeling fatigue, joint swelling, rashes, and sensitivities of unknown origins. Taking on a lot of responsibilities, worrying about them, and having the need to fulfill society's expectations can become a chronic stressor for you and may manifest in your physical body when uncared for.

Letting go of the past trauma and emotional baggage will help ease the burden the body is carrying. You could be carrying these for years and not even realize it. You have not fully let them go and have been dragging them along with you, picking up more load along the way. In time, they can weigh you down, and you can collapse from exhaustion. Your body may one day not be able to sustain your lifestyle and can start to break down.

You have to first recognize what the burdens are that are weighing you down and where they are stored in your body and start to release them emotionally, physically, energetically, and spiritually.

Although your past is a stepping stool for your own growth, the lingering effects that are not needed in your life at present can be carried over when left unchecked. You were so busy surviving and taking care of obligations and caring for everyone else that you never really took the time to filter what you had been through and what you took with you along your journey. Some things are necessary, such as virtue, honesty, resilience, and faith, but the negative or harmful habits that you have picked up need to be let go, such as holding grudges, being unable to forgive, biting your tongue and holding out on speaking your truth including disregarding your own needs and comfort as second to others.

Each person learns lessons and picks up baggage as they journey in life. It all depends which ones created an impact in their life, whether it be trauma or lessons learned. The more you hold on to the things you do not need, the things that harm and do not benefit you, the more it stagnates. You need to know what to keep and what to let go.

It can become a challenge to sift through all of these when they have become ingrained as a habit. A habit is a way of doing something over and over again, constantly and repeatedly, such that it eventually becomes an unconscious, effortless response. It becomes second nature to you. It will not be easy for you to see your habits clearly because it has now become a norm and has assimilated as normal in your everyday life. It could possibly take you a lot of time to see this, but you can also choose to ask for help if you want to facilitate your process.

When I first saw Kate on the other side of the screen during our online session, I saw a beautiful bright soul who could light up a room and light up people's lives. She had a stunning, radiant smile and a beautiful face with natural gorgeous hair. As I cleared the energy through sound vibration, I saw deeper and connected more clearly with where she was at that moment. I felt my heart start to palpitate, and the pulsation started to spread throughout my arms and my whole body. Without thinking, I heard myself say, "Kate, do you, by any chance, have some hypertension or high blood pressure?" She immediately replied with surprise, "How did you know?" There was a certain kind of vibration and frequency that felt stuck on her chest area that felt heavy. Kate was a very giving person, always striving to bring brightness, light, and love to those she met, especially those who she felt needed it the most. She liked to maintain harmony, disliked discord, and always tried to make others feel better. She was loving by nature but nowadays found herself tired, sad, and lonely. She tried to be good to herself but had a challenge in putting her needs ahead of others.

Kate is a forty-year-old mother of three, each child from a different father. She was unmarried, loyal, loving, and gave her all in each of her relationships. She never wanted things to end with the fathers of her children, and even though some of her exes remained good friends with her, she often wondered why things didn't work out. She desired to have the ideal happy family life, married with the man of her dreams, and nurturing her lovely children in a loving home. There was a sadness and loneliness deep in her that needed to be addressed and acknowledged.

In our following session, we worked on emotional mapping, also known as brain mapping. Through this map, one can find the origin of a conflict or patterns of energies, emotions, actions, and reactions that may hinder one's goals. It can bring to light the unconscious mind and the energetic currents that are residing in the body. Sometimes people think they are where they are, but in reality, they are really not. It is like a mirage or being in the movie *The Matrix*. Things may seem clear in your perspective at present, and you've always believed them to be the truth, but in reality, they are far from it. Someone comes along and snaps you into your actual reality. These are those "Aha!" moments when someone mirrors your true self back to you. Acknowledging these conscious and unconscious parts of us can lead to healing and acceptance of self, thereby creating a space to be empowered to live our authentic life.

During the session with Kate, I picked up on the word "abuse:" self-abuse vs. self-love. So we started working from there. At age seven, she was a shy and quiet child. She remembered being a good girl who liked and needed praises. She remembered that she loved her father for being supportive despite his being abusive to her mother. Her parents continued to stay together and her father was the "man" figure in Kate's life. Kate remembered that all she ever wanted was love in her home life.

At fourteen years old, she felt troubled and unwanted. She started looking for love. She ran away and had her first sexual experience, wherein she became pregnant. Her mother, knowing of her situation, aided her through abortion. She felt that she had no choice and went through with the abortion. Through her storytelling, I started to hear/feel children's voices, and a clear message came through: blame. I guided Kate through her experience, and she worked out that unconsciously she blamed herself for going through the abortion. She said that she blamed herself for all those children who could have been born but did not get a chance to be in this world because of her action. I felt that this was the first time she really faced this truth and acknowledged this side of her.

At seventeen, Kate's memory of her time was sadness. She had her first child with someone she loved, named Mark, who in her eyes was the "man" figure in her life. She enjoyed being with Mark and showered Mark and her first child with all of her heart and affection. She said that initially Mark was very supportive, but later on, he somehow felt trapped. From her memory, Kate's own father was happy for her and supportive of her decision to bring up a child at a young age. Her mother, however, was upset that she had gotten pregnant again.

At eighteen years old, Kate moved out of her parent's house, and when she was twenty-one, she and Mark broke up. They had been together for about six years. Afterwards, Kate met Rob, who was physically attractive, responsible, and caring. She had good chemistry and a spiritual connection with Rob. They had a child together when Kate was twenty-four years old, but Kate eventually called it quits and left Rob despite Rob's love for her. She started feeling guilty that she was not being fair to Rob. Rob adored her, but Kate was looking for something else—the "man" figure, which she did not see in Rob. Although their partnership did not last, she and Rob remained friends to this day.

When Kate was thirty-three years old, she was in a relationship with a man named Tony. He used Kate's financial stability and her emotional and energetic space to love and care in order to fulfill his needs. At thirty-four, Kate became pregnant with her third child. She said that her children were her happiness, and she loved getting pregnant and having children. This was a sense of escape for her, a safe space to love an innocent human being. She enjoyed being the nurturer. Congruently, it also brought to light that she used pregnancy as a crutch to be loved and to hold on to the relationship she had with most of the men in her life. She felt that having a child with them would make them stay for good. At this point in her life, she also started feeling depressed. She started feeling sad, tired, and lonely. This is when she started to look for ways to help herself and this is how she came to find me at the time that she needed. This comes back to: coincidences are not merely coincidences. When it is aligned, what you need will present itself. It is up to you to take action or non-action.

Working with Kate, I helped her realize that she was looking for that "man" figure. As with the law of attraction, this is what she was attracting and was attracted to. So the cycle repeated, and she did not know why it kept repeating and why she kept falling for the same type of "man." In her belief, the meaning of love for her was someone who could be happy for her, be supportive, but could also be abusive. In her mind, abuse was part of showing love. This was her belief of what a "man" figure was, similar to her experience growing up with her father and seeing how her father was to her mother. She also came to understand why she was not ready for Rob, who seemed to be the perfect man for her at the time to be able to give her what she wanted.

The relationship with her mother was also brought to light where guilt and blame was involved with the abortion. Kate stated that every time she became pregnant, her mother got upset. This was actually an epiphany that this was her mother's way of showing that she cared and loved Kate. Her mother did not want Kate to bring up children of her own at a very young age or all on her own as her mother could see how difficult this would be for Kate.

Kate is now working on attracting the right kind of man she wants for her life and learning to navigate on who and what the right man is for her. She is working on giving herself a voice to say NO when her heart says NO. She does not need to engage in a sexual relationship when she is not ready just to fulfill the need of her man so that he will stay in the relationship. He does not deserve to be in her life if he does not respect her. That is not the "man" she is looking for anymore. I helped her realize that she is important enough and deserves to be loved. She is working on what self-love means for her. Kate now sees her patterns and habits and is prepared to face and recognize them when they come. This will give her the space to make a choice of continuing in that pattern or create a change for herself.

Throughout our sessions, unknowingly, Kate kept on sighing out deeply, especially when realizations came to her. As I felt her energy become clearer and brighter, her chest also became lighter. Hope was stemming from her own life experiences. She was now able to distinguish between her habits and patterns and where she wanted to be in her life.

Your past can bleed into your present. It can even affect your physical health. You may be feeling such symptoms like palpitations, a pit in your stomach, holding your breath, or discomfort in your body that can be related to holding on to the energies of your past. It can even affect the way you think, the way you make decisions, and the way you do things. It is a major factor in forming your personality and your habits. Therefore, if your past has this effect, then that means that your present can do the same for your future. When this happens, it is important to prepare yourself to face your past. This can show you where the blockages you have placed within yourself and what impacted you the most that could be the reason stopping you from moving forward in your life.

The past has already happened. You cannot turn back time and change things that happened in the past. The present, however, gives you many chances and opportunities to create the basis of your future. If you want to form humility or compassion as a part of your character, you can start practicing that in the now until you build and grow that trait into a habit of effortlessly being a part of your life.

Forgiveness and acceptance are needed to move forward from your past. This means that you need to fully face and embrace the most impactful and the most uncomfortable events of your life that are difficult for you to bring up, especially the ones you always want to avoid, the ones that are most painful. Be thankful and honored to have the opportunity to grow and a chance to move forward, learning how to free yourself from your own preconceptions and limitations. Do not limit yourself in being the best version of you.

You may have not been conscious or aware of your life as it was unfolding in the past, but at present, you can now be aware or conscious of it. Awareness of the present, along with mindfulness and a connection to your heart and soul are the start to growth and healing. Through this, you can heal yourself to your completeness if you choose to take action toward it. You can reach your optimal well-being.

Chapter 11
Obstacles—Beliefs

"I want to be healthy, but no matter what I do, why is my situation not changing and just seems to be getting worse? I keep thinking and praying to become healthy, but why is it not happening?" This talks about the law of attraction.

What I have found is that you need to be ready for what you want. You need to be ready for what you are asking for. For instance, you want to have abundance of money, and you try different businesses or work more jobs, but you are unhappy, and somehow it is not enough or it does not work out. You need to ask what blockage or beliefs you have that are hindering you from manifesting what you want. The deeper you search, you may find that you are actually not ready or have a fear about having too much money. You may have a belief that the more money you have, the more problems you may have or that people who have a lot of money are not good people and look down on those who have less than them. You may not think this is true of you, but the more you are honest with yourself, you will know which is the real truth and which is your pretend truth. This belief and fear you have can be your own blockage from the flow of abundance. You are not fully ready to embrace it. What you actually truthfully believe is what is showing up in your reality. Knowing what is blocking you can facilitate in removing the blockage and letting abundance flow.

Think of when you asked God to help you be accepted in that job interview of your dreams, and you went to the interview and did not get it. You get other jobs easily but not your dream job. You have tried many times but someone else gets it. You may find later on that what was stopping you is that deep down, even though it may be your dream job, you actually believe that you are not good enough for that job, and you unconsciously feel that you are not ready for it yet. You may feel overwhelmed with the responsibility and allow fear to hinder your dream. So, in reality, you actually receive what you truly believe in and not what you think you are ready for.

In my case, when it came to my health, I realized that I did not give value and importance on the other aspects of myself. I only focused on making my physical body feel better, not fully believing that my energy body, emotions, thoughts, and spirit body were all related to my overall well-being. This I learned reflected on my physical body. I realized that I needed to give equal importance in taking care of all aspects of me.

Once you face this truth, you can start to unblock yourself from your own preconceptions and limitations. You align your priorities and what you really want in your life. Once the blockage clears, then the flow of the universe is in your hands. Things will fall into place and what you truly and sincerely ask for will come to reality.

Similarly, this applies to your physical body's condition. Why is it that even if I follow the doctor, eat what I am supposed to eat, avoid what needs to be avoided, drink vitamins, and try to live a healthy lifestyle,

I still feel horrible and have all kinds of aches, pains, and discomfort? You may have a belief that only medical doctors have the authority to help you. You may not want to look into the other aspects of yourself. That may be a fear of finding out more about yourself or fear of facing yourself.

If you know that there are many aspects of your body that can affect your physical body, then what is stopping you from finding out where the blockage is? What belief do you have that is blocking you from healing when you feel that you are desperately wanting to heal?

People say they want to change, but they are actually not ready to change, so they choose not to do anything, and so nothing changes. They then complain that nothing's changed.

We are actually the ones who create most of our roadblocks in life. Our own preconceptions and limiting beliefs can hinder us from the success, healing, and fulfillment that we are looking for. Acknowledging this and moving to learn more about yourself and growing yourself can help with unblocking and resuming the flow of life that you are authentically meant to live.

Healing takes time. True. How much time? It all depends. Growing up, society expects us to take plenty of time to grieve. It is important to process your emotions well. However, it is a misconception that healing always takes a very long time. When you understand what is needed for healing to take place and take action toward it, the healing process is facilitated. On the other hand, the more you do not want to face it, avoid it, and ignore it, the more it stays in your body. It is the unfinished business that needs to be worked out.

Healing needs to go through its process. Everyone has their own way of processing and healing. The time for healing and moving forward does not need to have a set time frame. Society appears to have made an accepted belief that if you care for and love someone deeply, you are expected to mourn longer for their loss, whether it be through death, debilitating illness, a breakup, or just being apart. If your healing was too short, it means you did not really love them that much. This I found to be a misconception.

The healing process can take longer when you hold on and are not able to let go of the reality of the situation. It is holding on to that attachment to that person. It also takes a toll on your body when it is being ignored or not being able to fully process. You may want to show that you are a pillar of strength, someone to trust and lean on, so you pretend that you are for others when in reality, you are not. You put aside your grieving process or you cut it short because you might feel that you need to move on and care for everyone else. They need you, so you say to yourself, "I need to be the one who is strong. I need to show strength. I can't keep wallowing in sorrow when my kids need me, when my younger siblings need me, when my family needs me." You ignore your own needs and your own healing. This, in the long run, can be a burden that you will be carrying. You put it aside in the attic of your body and it will not resolve itself unless it is addressed.

You may even choose to not share what you are going through with your kids or family because you do not want them to worry or want them to be burdened. You do not want them to carry any burden at all or be hurt. You would rather carry it all. Your kids are your life, and you would carry all their burdens for them as much as you possibly can. So you try to protect your loved ones, unknowingly hurting yourself and not allowing them to grow into their own experience.

I find it best to be truthful about how you are feeling, sharing with your loved ones as they most likely are going through their own healing process. Healing together creates a stronger bond. Speaking from the heart and speaking the truth is the key to effective communication. Always speak from truth and speak from a space of love. Say, "I am angry because I feel I have no control over the situation. There is nothing I can do," or, "I feel very sad and in a lot of hurt because I lost someone I love. It hurts even when I know that he/she is in a better place." This is acknowledging your truth. Facing your truth is a sign of growth and healing.

Healing takes place when you decide to face your own pain. Courage is not only facing your fears but allowing yourself to fully process the pain that comes along with it. It is okay to face your pain. It is then that you will find clarity. You may want to bargain and go back to how things were, back to your comfort zone, but there will be no progress. Growth happens when you fully embrace all of you, including all your feelings even if it can be borderline unbearable. It is you who generated that pain, which means that it is also you who can help heal that pain.

> *"Pain is a part of life. It is when we*
> *experience pain that we grow the most."*

Balance in a relationship is loving yourself enough to love someone else. However, this can sometimes hurt too. We tend to buy material things to show we love someone. It makes us happy, buying things for our love ones. We want to make our loved ones feel special, cared for, and loved. Although that can be true, overdoing this may cause materialism. When I say materialism, I mean the value one person puts in a material thing becomes more than the pureness of the intention itself.

The giving of material things is not the only way to show your love. It is felt more through your mindful and caring ways, like offering someone tea or coffee when they had a long day at work or even relaxing or giving them a hug when they need it the most. You take care of them when they are sick, supporting them when they are in a rush, helping them with what they need. Those little things mean more than any material value. You created an energetic space of comfort, security, and a feel good state. You should do the same for your own self. You are deserving of it. Having the sincere respect for yourself gives you a space to also see others and give them respect.

Along the way, if things do not work out, because sometimes they do not, you have the capacity to know what true love really is, even when it hurts immensely. You will learn not to give up on your own values and dreams for someone else, and you will choose not to hold back the dreams of your loved one as well, even when you both desperately want your relationship to work. Love can sometimes be bittersweet, and it also includes learning when to let go and set each other free.

Real love means sometimes letting go no matter how much it hurts. You will know what true love really means. You will find that love knows no bounds. It is important to address any obstacle, misunderstanding, or blockages in a relationship. If you feel you easily irritate each other for little reasons, that needs to be brought to light because there can be hidden issues that have been buried or ignored. It is important to value truth over pain. Truth is important because living a lie with yourself is a heavy burden for your body to bear.

When your growth is stagnant, when life is stagnant and sluggish, it can cause depression or boredom. It can cause you to live like a zombie, going through the motions of the day not fully living. This often happens when we disregard our needs over others or society's expectations. Do not give up your dream for someone else's. Allow your dream to come true. It is then that you can say that you are truly living—your spirit alive, awake, and in charge.

Go through the motions of healing, embrace the pain, run through your doubts, blame, and guilt, and choose growth and healing through it all. You will find that one day, perhaps sooner than you expect, you are ready to move forward in your life. In grief, the memories are most painful. But through healing, you will find that those same memories will one day become celebrated, honored, and enjoyed. They will become not painful but your happy memories.

The physical body is only temporary. This is reality. We, as humans, will go through birth, growth, and eventually death. It is normal, and everyone will go through it. I want to talk about this because I feel that it is really important to face our mortality, especially when you reach a certain age. Most older adults begin to prepare for their end of life, and that is totally alright. They may have hired a lawyer for their last will and testament. They may have purchased land where they would like to be buried. They may even be looking for nursing homes, group homes, or assisted living for their last years on earth.

For many of you, you may be dreading facing this. You dread being the cause of hardship and pain to your family. In truth, you dread getting older and have difficulty accepting this reality. You believe that you will naturally get sick, get dementia, and be unable to care for yourself. The more you truly believe this, the higher the possibility that you will manifest it in reality. You may feel that this is your only future as this is what everyone else seem to be going through, this is the trend and what seems to be the norm.

In this day and age, the average lifespan has increased. We are in an era of advancement in all fields where we are given the capacity to live longer. If so, then why start packing your bags from living? I say, create your own reality, your own future, how you want to go out from this world, how you want to live your life until your last breath. You can choose not to live like a zombie going through life conforming to what society expects and what you expect of yourself. Live life to the fullest and complete your mission and life's dream until your very last day on earth. I believe that until our last breath, we are given all that time to live out our life's purpose and to live our grandest self.

I remember the time when I had worked with a loving couple who had been husband and wife for a long time, Jonathan and Faith. Jonathan had to retire earlier than he'd like to due to his slowly-worsening fine motor skills. His hands and fingers would sometimes shake uncontrollably. They had seen specialists to help with his condition but did not know if his situation would get better or would worsen. Faith put all her time, energy, and effort in helping Jonathan, the love of her life, in getting better and was slowly getting frustrated, desperate, and borderline exhausted. Faith saw that Jonathan needed help with many activities of daily living. She wanted to know if I could see whether Jonathan would get better or if she needed to prepare for the worst.

Now, I am not one to predict anyone's future, as I believe that is not my place. I assess the present, and we work from there. I could not give Faith the answer that she wanted to hear, but I saw an energetic imbalance between them. There was a moment when Jonathan needed to adjust his belt when Faith was about to help him that I encouraged to give him the space to have him take care of himself. Jonathan said, "I can do it," and he did without much difficulty. We did exercises for clearing and cleansing, gathering and accumulating energy. I guided them through sharing that energy, circulating between the two of them. I wanted them to experience and feel for themselves that sharing their energy together and nurturing each other's strength and love, is what makes them stronger to create the change they have always dreamed of. They experienced fully that moment of being in that bubble of safety, love and affection, solidifying their unit as a whole. After the exercise, Jonathan, who was emitting radiant and pure energy, who worried less about his condition, said that this is what he had wanted to share with Faith. They obviously love each other and want to ease each other's burdens. He knew all the things Faith had done for him and how much she loves him. He always wanted to give back. Faith was so focused on Jonathan's well-being that she forgot how to receive. She needed to really embrace and fully receive all of Jonathan's love as well. There was a shift in their energy and a shift in their physical bodies by the end of the session. It almost felt like their bodies just took a sigh, a breath of release. Sometimes, trying to control a situation beyond our control due to fear can cause blockages. Our thought of "My loved one needs me. I need to be strong and keep it together for his sake" can easily go down a path of self-neglect—others first, before myself. When we deplete ourselves, we can start to feel unease of the body and predispose ourselves to being ill.

I encouraged them to exercise what I had showed them, to allow Jonathan to be a little more independent, and reminded Faith that she did not have to be alone in taking on everything. She needed to remind herself to fully receive the love Jonathan had been always willing and wanting to share with her. She was so focused in her own care for him that she did not give him room to share his love for her. He was not as weak or helpless as she thought he was. In his own way, he could also take care of her and provide for what she needed, which was love. After the exercises, they talked about the house they had just bought in California but also had thoughts of moving and purchasing another house in Nevada. I mentioned how there was something about this house in California they recently bought that was significant to them as a couple. Faith finally shared with me that it had been a dream of theirs to get this house in California, design, and renovate it together in the way that fit their lifestyle. There was a hint of a spark when talking about their dream project together as a couple. They had obviously put this dream in the backburner because of Faith's worry about Jonathan.

We know our physical body changes as we grow older, but this alone should not stop us from continuing on to make our dreams a reality. Following your heart and going for your dreams can help boost your energy and brighten your spirit. It can make you feel alive and full of life. Where did that vitality come from? It came from your soul. It came from within you. Grow your spirit to be strong. Our physical body may one day pass, but the spirit lives on. A balance in taking care of your health, managing your energy, following your heart, and going for your dreams is important. I know it is easier said than done. But it is through sincere commitment, practice, and mindful actions that we can find what balance is for us.

You can do what you always wanted to do, find what lights the fire of passion in your heart. Write a bucket list of things you want to do and places you want to go before your physical body passes away in this world. It is never too late to start anything, no matter your age or status.

We will all go through death. That's reality. Go and live without regrets until your last breath. Be your own inspiration. When you inspire yourself, you are also impacting and inspiring your loved ones. Find out if this is how you would rather want your future to be.

You get to have a choice in your future. Right here, right now, you have that choice, you have that power over your life. Whatever your circumstance is right now, choice is your superpower. Choice is your God-given right. Use it well.

Living a life filled with many responsibilities, especially if they are mainly not focused on your own and focused on the well-being of others instead, can cause you to lose energy and lose a part of yourself. Putting others first ahead of your own self or taking on society's beliefs that do not speak true to your heart can cause a discrepancy in your own life when they do not align with your truth.

I remember a time when I had been restless, having a lot of interests. I would often be enthusiastic in the beginning and later on lose interest and end up not finishing projects that I started. I would go about the humdrum of life: work, school, family, gym/yoga. I was stable financially and physically healthy. But when I saw myself in the mirror, looked into my own eyes, I saw lifeless dead fish eyes staring right back at me. I asked myself, "What happened to you?" When I look at photos of myself growing up, I can see where the light in my eyes started to dim. There is a saying that the eyes are the window to the soul. I do believe that in a way this is true. I did see my soul stashed somewhere in the back collecting dust. I did not give it space to grow and be free. I said to myself in the mirror, "What happened to you? Why are you dead? We have to figure out how to get you back out in the open."

I tried many things like yoga, meditation, joining religious events and choir, attending mass more regularly, going to the gym, spending more time with people I cared about. I went to many trainings for self-growth and healing. I moved about in nursing units and even travelled all over the world. I realized I actively started seeking living alive again, looking to grow that spark. Somehow, I lost the spark of life and that realization prompted me to search. "Ask and you shall receive," Jesus from the Bible said. You need to do your part and be ready to receive. Just like in a river, the fresh water comes to you from the snow on the mountaintops. It flows through the river to reach you. If there was a blockage in that river that is blocking the flow and you do nothing, you do not choose to take action to remove that blockage, then that fresh water from the mountaintops may never arrive to you. On the other hand, when you remove the blockage, the river will flow and fresh, natural, clean water comes along, but if you are not ready to gather the water, you can miss your chance and not receive what you have asked for. You have to actively ask, actively search, and actively receive.

Congruently, the belief that "Jesus is my Savior" applies if you actively live it. Many people say this yet choose to drink too much alcohol, eat what they are not supposed to, speak unkindly, think unlovingly, try to manipulate or control others, or put too much burden on themselves like blame and shame. There is a parable in the Bible found in Matthew 25:14-30 called *A Story About Three Servants*. It says,

"The kingdom of heaven is like a man who was going to another place for a visit. Before he left, he called for his servants and told them to take care of his things while he was gone. He gave one servant five bags of gold, another servant two bags of gold, and a third servant one bag of gold, to each one as much as he could handle. Then he left. The servant who got five bags went quickly to invest the money and earned five more bags. In the same way, the servant who had two bags invested them and earned two more. But the servant who got one bag went out and dug a hole in the ground and hid the master's money."

"After a long time the master came home and asked the servants what they did with his money. The servant who was given five bags of gold brought five more bags to the master and said, 'Master, you trusted me to care for five bags of gold, so I used your five bags to earn five more.' The master answered, 'You did well. You are a good and loyal servant. Because you were loyal with small things, I will let you care for much greater things. Come and share my joy with me.'

"Then the servant who had been given two bags of gold came to the master and said, 'Master, you gave me two bags of gold to care for, so I used your two bags to earn two more.' The master answered, 'You did well. You are a good and loyal servant. Because you were loyal with small things, I will let you care for much greater things. Come and share my joy with me.'

"Then the servant who had been given one bag of gold came to the master and said, 'Master, I knew that you were a hard man. You harvest things you did not plant. You gather crops where you did not sow any seed. So I was afraid and went and hid your money in the ground. Here is your bag of gold.' The master answered, 'You are a wicked and lazy servant! You say you knew that I harvest things I did not plant and that I gather crops where I did not sow any seed. So you should have put my gold in the bank. Then, when I came home, I would have received my gold back with interest.'

"So the master told his other servants, 'Take the bag of gold from that servant and give it to the servant who has ten bags of gold. Those who have much will get more, and they will have much more than they need. But those who do not have much will have everything taken away from them.' Then the master said, 'Throw that useless servant outside, into the darkness where people will cry and grind their teeth with pain.'"

It is like in this parable that we should honor, care, nurture and grow what God, who is the source, has entrusted us with. We are entrusted with the tools to grow these bags of gifts and talents. These tools include our physical and energy body, our thoughts, and our emotions. Growing our gifts involves growing the character of our spirit. This involves taking care of all aspects of our body—our mind, body, energy, and spirit. It is important to be aware of what we put our body through, what our body is telling us, and mindful of our thoughts and actions because they are in connection to what our spirit really wants. Find a balance of having a loving and healthy relationship with all aspects of your being.

The more you grow bigger, brighter, and stronger with the gifts and talents that were given to you, the more you have the capacity to impact many people's lives, the more you can help and the more you can serve. Our physical and energy body gives us the ability to share these gifts and talents; therefore, it is equally important to care for our physical and energy body in order to share our spirit.

Honoring God is not trying to convince someone else that your religion is better than others. It is taking good care of all God has entrusted you with, growing and sharing the gifts and talents that are given to you, including taking care of humanity and the earth that God has provided us to nurture. Share with loving intention. It is through you, your actions, and your life that people will know and learn what love is—the love who is the God in you and through you.

There is a saying, "If you don't use it, you lose it." The same as in the parable. If you do not grow your gifts or talents, they can become rusty and unusable. If you become stuck, stagnant, blocked, and unmoving for growth, then you may eventually lose what you were given and the capacity to fulfill your dreams. You're unable to fulfill your life's mission because you have not developed the tools and talents needed to accomplish it. Your life can lose its sense of purpose. Unknowingly for many, this leads to depression.

I grew up Catholic, very devout, as was expected of me. At the same time, I am also partially Chinese and also lived with Oriental culture. What I disliked with religion growing up was seeing the discrepancy of claiming or showing that you are prayerful but treating people unkindly and being hurtful. It was a form of power. Intuitively, I knew it wasn't the way it should be, but this is why I believe that it does not matter what religion a person is, but what matters more is how you treat people. For me, religion is a guide on how to live your life well and how you should treat each other. It defeats the purpose when you show up and do not practice what you supposedly believe in. I'm not saying everyone is like this. But I have seen others who are not Catholic who treat people better than those who are. It is very hypocritical, I had said at the time. This is why it is important to also clearly see what your truth is and know what you're all about.

At a really young age, I just knew certain things that I chose not to believe in and to be against what was told of me. It was only as I grew older that I ended up listening more to the majority than myself. This is why it is really important to allow our loved ones to grow into their own real selves, nurture and support their life's missions, rather than imposing our own reality on them. They have the ability to know what is right and what is wrong. That needs to be reinforced in their upbringing. They need to find their own way, not always being told step-by-step what to do, but come to find out what their life's purpose is and support that.

I used to believe in coincidence or luck. Now, I realize that we can create our own luck. Luck does happen, but the will and conviction to action are what moves things to come to reality. Life is never a coincidence. I used to take for granted many messages from life, and in a way, I felt that I had neglected my own self. I eventually started to believe what everybody else believed because I had gotten used to it and it was easier. But I saw that I was slowly dying inside, and I do not want to live life like a walking, talking zombie. Whenever I find that spark of life, I will live with it for a little bit, then go back to being a zombie again. Many times, I was not aware when I had reverted back to zombieism. That's a word I made up. Zombieism—the act of living life like a zombie—a walking, talking lifeless, emotionless, heartless living-dead person.

I had been in and out of zombieism but never gave up. I later on found the reason for feeling this way. It was that the connection to my soul needed to be stronger. I had been told what to do, what is right, what needs to be done, what to believe, but deep down, I was really not convinced that all of these were my truth. I was not brought up to grow my own intuition, which was very strong as a child. My intuition went against what was considered the norm and the expected. I started to listen and believe others more than believing in myself, my inner voice, my soul. Your intuition is the unexplainable, irrational part of you that somehow just adds up to be just exactly what you need in your life. There is no explanation for it, but it just fits perfectly. You feel it makes sense and feels right even if rationally it does not make sense. This part of you needs to be cultivated and listened to because intuition has a direct connection to your soul. It is your soul's message, your soul's voice.

In zombieism, you become numb and apathetic, and you do not even realize when you are hurt or when there is a cut or a wound on your body. You do not feel it anymore. Either that, or you are too busy focusing on others and you do not feel what is being inflicted on your own self. This is when all the things you are carrying or holding in your body, all the scars and wounds in your body, are being ignored. As your body has its own healing abilities, in the long run, it is unable to sustain your own homeostasis. It tries so hard to keep up with you and your lifestyle, your way of life—emotionally, mentally, physically, and spiritually. You will only pay attention to it when it becomes unbearable or when it shows up as a life-altering situation. This most often comes up as illness in physical form. It is only then do you start to pay attention.

It is because I chose to never give up in growing my spirit to be brighter that I learned to keep choosing to live fully alive and come out of zombieism. The reason I had kept on reverting back to zombieism is because it had been ingrained so much that it became my habit, a part of my life. I spent a lot of money and a lot of my time to grow myself, to have my soul show up and be the driver of my life. Many times, my family tells me I wasted money on a lot of these things that they do not see value in. I knew somehow; I did not regret any of it. Your search may lead you to know that one thing may not be for you, but most times, what shows up is exactly what you need. You just need to show up, be present, and move to take action.

In time, I noticed that I had started to doubt my own intuition because of all the other outside noise and information I took on and believed over my own. Unconsciously, I had slowly and gradually muted my own inner voice. This is why I could not hear it clearly. And since it is my soul's voice, I had silenced it. This is why I was unhappy and living as a zombie. It was when I made the choice in growing the real me that things turned around for me.

As society often dictates how we should live our life, we think that working hard and saving a lot of money for the future is the key to happiness. You work too hard and too much, have the money, and by the time you retire, you have the money and the time, but you do not have the physical capacity to do the things you wanted to do in the first place. There needs to be a balance between what you want and what is needed.

In the Bible, the Gospel of Matthew 7:7-8 says, "Ask, and God will give you. Search, and you will find. Knock, and the door will open for you. Yes, everyone who asks will receive. Everyone who searches will find. And everyone who knocks will have the door opened."

This quote does not mean you do nothing. I'm going to give this example: When you want something to eat, know what you want. For instance, you want vegetables. This is the Ask. You are not able to get these vegetables when you do not look or search to find out where the supermarket is. This is the Search. You do not get these vegetable when you do not step out of the house to go to the supermarket to buy them. This is the Knock. What you are asking for is provided. It is up to you to do your part.

Also, be aware that whatever you ask for may not come in the exact form you expect but may come in another form. Open your eyes and mind to the messages. Trust and have faith that this is what is meant to happen. Everything works out in the end the way it should.

The law of attraction is related to manifestations to reality. When you want something badly but you actually do not believe it possible to happen, then it will most likely not come true. For example, when you want to be successful and you work hard, you try all kind of ways to be successful, but nothing seems to work, only to find out later on that your belief about success is actually a fear, the fear of taking on the responsibilities that come along with success. This fear is the block on the flow of your success.

Because of how you grew up, you may feel that you owe a lot to those who have helped you. You worked hard and made your own decisions to be in a space of abundance, having more than before, and now, you are made responsible to take care of those who have helped you. This is a great way of sharing your gifts and abundance. However, there needs to be a balance. You do not need to feel obligated to do something that is not in connection to your heart. You may feel the need and responsibility, but you also have to first take care of you. If you give away all of you and do not give or leave some for yourself, then you can be depleted.

When you give, you should not give that person the obligation to give back to you later on in life. The real gift of giving is not expecting anything in return. I remember a time when I gave my best friend stickers along with a notebook on her birthday. A few days later, she gave me a notebook along with stickers similar to the ones I gave her. It felt nice, but it didn't feel quite right either because I felt like she needed to give me back a favor.

You need to love yourself enough and give yourself the credit of making the choice to change your poorness to abundance, your hardship to comfort and security. Wanting to give back is great as long as it is healthy. Do not feel like you owe your entire life, your energy, and your money to the people who helped you in the past just because they supported you that one or few times so you can reach your goal.

Think of it this way: If they were unable to help you at the time you needed help and if you really want to reach your goal, you would have found another way. It did not have to be them. You are the one who did whatever was necessary to get to your goal to have a better life. You need to acknowledge that and see that you are the reason why you are where you are right now. People helped you along the way, and yes, it is good to show them your appreciation. But, you do not need to give them your life's work. You do not owe them your life energy. It is you who made the difference. You did it! Rejoice in that, and give yourself the credit you deserve.

You may think that you do not have a choice, but you do! That is something you always have that is yours alone. You might say, "I am but a small portion of the population; I will not need to do anything because it will not make a difference anyway. Those in power or position are the only ones who can make a difference." I say bull! This is simply not true. I used to believe this and have lived a passive life, going with the flow, accepting hopelessness in some aspects of life, admitting defeat, and just going along with what everyone else is doing. I know this now to be not true. Be aware of what may dim your light inside of you. It is most often the acceptance of defeat or choosing to hide your true nature by just going with the flow. Dimming the lights can be equivalent to slowly dying inside, a loss of power, a depletion of energy. Find that spark, and reignite your own flame. You can always choose this instead.

I remember a few times when I had been bold enough to not care what others thought and live out of my own truth. When I was in high school, I would speak of the elephant in the room and just asked direct questions, dressed the way I wanted, walked the way I walked, and spoke half English and half Ilonggo, a Filipino dialect. Many students befriended me, but I found out that some spoke about me behind my back. Some did not like the way I dressed because I did not dress like them, did not like the way I walked because I was told that I walked with confidence, and did not like the way I spoke because it made me seem superior to them. I was hurt when I found out. I had a talk with myself and tried to find out if I was the one who was wrong. It hurts to know that you opened yourself up to people and they judged you. I cried all night and felt all alone. It was during this time that I felt closer to myself, knowing that I could choose not to live my life to the standard of others, knowing that I could never please everyone. People always have something to say, and all I can do is live my life well without hurting anyone. I found out later on that I was both criticized and admired at the same time. I got looks, and some others told me how brave I was and how they wished they could do the same but never would. It was a lonely road for a while, being unable to put trust on people, but I grew from the experience.

In a way, I learned to put trust back into my own self. I learned to enjoy spending alone time with me. I have fond memories when looking back on some dates I had with myself. It was in those moments that I found time of peace. Not long after, I allowed myself to open my heart again to people. Now, I can see how I did not give up on people precisely because I did not give up on me.

Don't give up! Find your light and grow it! Know that you are not alone! We are in this journey called life—together. I see you, because in a way, I am you!

Chapter 12
Conclusion

When we're just kids, we are like that brand new car that runs smoothly with no problems. With our body compared to a vehicle, as you drive this car, you may go through rough roads, pot holes, dirt and uneven terrains, or encounter black ice. You may go through a war zone, which causes scrapes, scratches, holes, or marks on the car. If you always drive through the safe and boring roads, there will be no challenge and less room to grow your driving skills.

Just like a car, our body needs rest so as not to overheat. Overdoing it can overheat and damage the engine. The car also has a yearly inspection. This is your yearly doctor's checkup. You have to be on top of the upkeep of your car, such as having the oil changed, tuning, and removing rust, blockages, and any unwanted things that are hindering the smooth flow of your engine. This is the everyday check in with yourself. You can see how this is similar to maintaining and taking care of your body.

As in the car, the engine is the core, the energy source to start and activate the car. The engine needs to be strong and powerful for the car to have the life force to move. Strengthening the core is strengthening the body. This will help you get to your destination.

Emotions are the tools to upgrade our car. If someone damages the back of your car, then you learn to put a rubber bumper in the back. If your car tires have been stolen, you may want to get a tire lock. If you received a parking ticket, you become more mindful when and where you park. You become more aware of your own driving and those on the road with you. You will learn how to drive skillfully in the highways of life. You will know how to navigate through roads with all kinds of drivers.

Meanwhile, the driver of the car is up to you. It could be your Ego, or it could be your truth. Where you want to go could be led by your limiting beliefs, or it could be led by the freedom of your soul. It is extremely important who you choose to drive your car because it will affect where you will end up. Allowing your soul's heart to shine is the road to a healing journey of peace within yourself.

Eventually, our physical body will stop working, as with the end of life for the car. This is the beauty and wisdom of mortality. We are given a set time to grow, and thus, we should grow accordingly. Our soul is eternal, but our physical body has a limited lifespan. Having a physical body gives us the opportunity to move forward in growing our soul.

Mortality gives us the drive to live well, live with quality, purpose, and intention. When we acknowledge our mortality as our teacher, there is no time to waste. With a deadline, it gives us more reason to be motivated to grow ourselves, connect with our soul, and live our life to the fullest.

"Take care of your body. Grow your soul. Live and love with no regrets."

In summary, the choice to fully and wholeheartedly commit to learning more about yourself will be met with many challenges and lessons. Life will try and get in your way, but your conviction will show you the way.

Conviction is your solid, firm, and strong certainty about something. Your conviction level depends on the strength of your mind and willpower. Be clear that this is absolutely what you want. Remember this moment—the moment of CHOOSING to COMMIT to knowing and growing yourself to a path of healing. Promise yourself that once you start on this path, turning back is not an option. Do not allow your own excuses to chain you down from living your 100%. Grow your conviction in loving yourself enough to invest in your own well-being.

Condition your mind to be ready for anything and everything. There are infinite possibilities in your healing process. Be present 100% right here, right now. Get to know your body intimately like a lover or a best friend. Be kind and compassionate toward yourself and know that mistakes are okay. Accept and acknowledge all you wish to improve. Be ready to meet with and have a close and loving relationship with your body and your mind, and let your spirit shine through.

When you sincerely commit to something, everything you need or ask for will effortlessly come to you. It will just be a matter of whether you do something about it or not. Be open and be aware that it may come as not what you expect, but when it appears, you will say, "Aha! You are exactly what I was looking for. Thank you!"

Trust that circumstances and the people that show up in your life are not just coincidences. Where you have been, what you have been through, the choices you've made, and the people that have impacted your life were all necessary for you to build your character. Those life skills and mind exercises helped you grow to be the person you are now, getting you ready to be the person you want to be. It is like gaining a superpower each time you overcome each obstacle. These superpowers are necessary for your growth and healing.

Stress is a necessary part of life. Although stress can be helpful to move us to growth, it can also be unhealthy when we are exposed to it for prolonged periods of time. It can cause tightness in one or more aspect of your physical, mental, and emotional bodies. Checking in on ourselves needs to become a habit as well as learning to manage stress well.

You need to be ready to face yourself honestly and confidently. Be ready to face your pain and discomfort, both physically and emotionally. Be ready to face your own Ego and your own limitations. Recognize the blockages you have placed on yourself that shackle your own growth. Learn the reason behind those blockages and work to unbind and unlock them.

The earth is your training ground to grow yourself and help others along the way. And the best way to help others is to love yourself first and foremost. It is important to know how to distinguish what the true meaning of loving yourself is. To do this means developing a sincere relationship with all aspects of yourself: your body, your mind, and your spirit.

Pain is a part of life. Many times in life, what we perceive as difficult or painful may just be what we need to grow to better ourselves or to find the path our soul is trying to show us to follow.

When chronic pain or illness, fatigue, and invisible illness show up, it can be a sign to upgrade your life. It can indicate a time for a change, a reminder to find the light and grow the light of our spirit. It can tell us that there is no time to waste. You need to be ready to create a shift in your life. It is a time that your body may be telling you, "Listen to me! I am showing you to listen in to know what makes you happy. I am letting you know that it is time for you to step up, be the person you so desperately want to be, and live the life you want to live." Your spirit has been crying, and your body is starkly showing you the condition of the imbalance between your mind, body, and spirt. In other words, it is the disconnect between what you truly want in your life, your actions, and how you've been living your life. It can be a reminder that it is time to take charge of your life, align yourself with your truth, and actually live it.

Getting to know yourself gives you wisdom in understanding others as well. Other than being in the path of your own healing, you can also be there for others' healing and growth. Life is a cycle. Whatever you put out is what comes back. We share the same earth and need to encourage each other to choose light, truth, and love. We each have it. Others may not know it, but that is something we need to nurture and cultivate. You always have a choice in how you want to be. Be your own hero. Be your own inspiration. When you can fully accept the all that is you, you can fully accept others. When others know that you accept them and love them for who they are, including the parts they abhor about themselves, healing already begins.

We are all here to help each other. Just because you feel like you are less healthy than others or less worthy than others does not mean that is the truth. When you learn your truth by being connected to your divine spirit, you know that you are enough. You are light. You are love. Just grow that and live that.

They say practice makes perfect. Heal your life, grow your soul, follow your heart, and help others along the way. You may trip and fall many times, and that is okay. The road to understanding and connection with your true self and the path to living the life you want in your optimum capacity are not only for a numbered few but are absolutely possible for you, me, and anyone and everyone choosing the journey toward that path.

Choose the life you want to live. Choose healing and growth. Commit to it, and take action. Clear your thoughts, and follow your heart. Be your own cheerleader, and follow through. Embrace love and all goodness. Celebrate yourself.

Live the life you are authentically meant to live.

Acknowledgments

Writing this book has been a humbling and healing experience for me. It was never an intention of mine to be an author, but a dream and my aunt's wisdom had encouraged me to write this book.

I want to thank God, foremost, the source, the universe, the encompassing, for all that is possible, for the connection and guidance in the process of writing this book and in the process of my being and my life.

Thank you to my sister, my beloved kindred spirit, who always knows what to say and was a perfect support during this whole process of writing and most especially in the growth of my life.

I also want to thank my soul family, Sedona Mago and Body and Brain, for helping me find a home where I can be understood and fully accepted in my growth and in all my eccentricities.

I am truly grateful for Angela Lauria. It was a dream message that led me to you, and now this book is a reality. Throughout the process of writing this book, a breakthrough in my life occurred. It gave me clarity that propelled me to be ready for the next chapter of my life. Thank you for the heart and the help that you are.

To my sweet fairy god-editor, Bethany Davis, thank you for sharing your heart and expertise in helping me make this book whole in its entirely. I am grateful for your patience, understanding, support, and encouragement. You are absolutely the perfect one to have helped me edit in this book journey.

To the Morgan James Publishing team: Special thanks to David Hancock, CEO & Founder for believing in me and my message. To my Author Relations Manager, Margo Toulouse, thanks for making the process seamless and easy. Many more thanks to everyone else, but especially Jim Howard, Bethany Marshall, and Nickcole Watkins.

Thank you to all my friends and family who have been active in supporting me and my life endeavors, most especially to Mustafa El Ouatyq, who has been instrumental in showing me my own strength and helping me see the conviction of my heart and the significance of my life's purpose. For Donna Kotoff, who has been the epitome of care and love, giving positive smiles and vibes to everyone she meets. For Maria Castillo, supermom and loyal superfriend, who is always happy for others' happiness. For Stephanie Murillo and Michelle Lin, my besties, who are more sisters than friends, thank you for your listening ears and encouraging hearts. I know I can always count on you for anything and everything.

I want to give thanks to those, here and there, who have made this book possible.

Thank you all for sharing your heart and for your never ending support.

And importantly, to you. Yes, you! The one who is reading this book. This book would be of no use without you. Thank you for giving this book life and purpose. I have written this book especially for you—

written from my heart to yours. May you be filled with love and wisdom and be empowered to live the life you want—with happiness, freedom, and your utmost well-being.

Love and light!

Marie Anne June L. Tagorda

Thank You!

Thank you so much for reading! The fact that you have gotten to this point is saying something: You're ready! You're ready to step up and take back your health and happiness.

As a thank you, I'm offering a bonus *Discerning Tool* I made especially for you to help start your journey into growth and healing. You can head to takingbackmyhealthbook.com to take the quiz and start your next steps.

About the Author

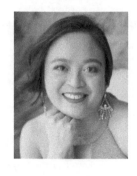

Marie Anne June L. Tagorda is a medical intuitive, energy healer, and spiritual intuitive adviser who specializes in releasing emotional trauma and healing the wounds of the past while rejuvenating the energetic connection between the mind, the body, and the heart.

As a critical care registered nurse and a life coach with a lifetime of experience as an oracle and intuitive healer, Marie Anne helps clients identify the root issues of their lives, bodies, minds, and spirits and helps them clear away the blockages that keep them from authentically living their best lives.

Her passion is to share humanity's innate nature of connectedness—connection to the internal and external world, connection with people and the natural earth.

Marie Anne completed Healer's School in Sedona from Body and Brain in 2007. She is also a Brain Management Consultant and a graduate of Power Brain Education. She received direct mentorship from award-winning author Rebecca Tinkle and manager of Sedona Healing Arts, Yolessa Lawrinnce for Spiritual Reading and Healing.

As a registered nurse since 2006, she has worked in a Medical Surgical Unit, Renal Unit, Respiratory Unit, Telemetry or heart monitoring Unit, the Surgical Intensive Care Unit, and the Post-Anesthesia Care Unit, also known as Recovery Room. She has seen the effects illness has on people and their loved ones and knew that she has the ability to be of more service additionally as a holistic integrative healer.

In New York, she discovered yoga in 2006 and has instructed energy-based yoga classes in her free time. She had also worked with children as a Power Brain Instructor.

She had searched for her life's purpose and found that helping with healing is what she is best at and is her soul's passion. She believes that as we heal ourselves, we heal the world.

Website: clearhealingmethod.com

Email: takingbackmyhealthbook@yahoo.com

Printed in the USA
CPSIA information can be obtained
at www.ICGtesting.com
JSHW082348140824
68134JS00020B/1951